SICK TO FIT

THREE SIMPLE TECHNIQUES THAT GOT ME
FROM 420 POUNDS TO THE COVER OF
RUNNER'S WORLD, GOOD MORNING
AMERICA, AND THE TODAY SHOW

JOSH LAJAUNIE

HOWARD JACOBSON, PHD

WellStart
Health

Da Fine Print

This book contains advice and information relating to health care. It should be used to supplement rather than replace the advice of your doctor or another health care professional. If you know or suspect that you have a health problem, it is recommended that you seek your physician's advice before embarking on any medical program or treatment.

All efforts have been made to assure the accuracy of the information contained in this book as of the date of publication. The publisher and the authors disclaim liability for any medical outcomes that may occur as a result of applying the methods suggested in this book.

Mentions of specific companies, organizations, or authorities in this book does not imply endorsement by the authors or publisher, nor does mention of specific companies, organizations, or authorities imply that they endorse this book, its authors, or the publisher. Internet addresses given in this book were accurate at the time it went to press.

PRAISE FOR SICK TO FIT

Raw and honest. Touching and motivating. Josh's path toward a healthy body and a healthful life is an inspiring and wonderful roadmap. Are you looking for transformation? Do you wish to make incredibly positive changes? Wish no more. This book is the practical guide.

— ROBERT OSTFELD, MD, MSc., DIRECTOR, PREVENTIVE CARDIOLOGY, MONTEFIORE HEALTH SYSTEM, AND ASSOCIATE PROFESSOR, MEDICINE, ALBERT EINSTEIN COLLEGE OF MEDICINE

Sick to Fit is a captivating, inspiring and practical story of an epic transformation. And don't be deceived by how entertaining this page-turner of a book is. What you're about to have fun reading is scientifically proven, and it just might change your life.

— OCEAN ROBBINS, AUTHOR, 31-DAY FOOD REVOLUTION, CEO, FOOD REVOLUTION NETWORK

A diet book with lots of information leaves you with lots of information. But a book that teaches you how to change your dietary and lifestyle habits – and do it in a way that is compelling, engaging, and eminently practical – a book like that can change your life.

Sick to Fit takes everything that we know about what makes people change in business and life, and applies it to eating and lifestyle habits. I've read a tremendous number of books on diet, fitness, and health - and this one is the best.

— PETER BREGMAN, AUTHOR, LEADING WITH EMOTIONAL
COURAGE, CEO, BREGMAN PARTNERS

One great and authentic story can move more hearts to change than all the book learning in the world. Josh's story has exactly that power to help so many join him in moving from *Sick to Fit*. I recommend you read it and follow the program which has proven to help so many reach their goals of better health and control.

— JOEL KAHN MD, FACC, AUTHOR, THE PLANT BASED
SOLUTION

Sick To Fit is chock-full of extraordinarily simple, realistic and common sense advice that will have you enthusiastically nodding your head while wondering why the hell you didn't come up with these ideas on your own. It spells out in no uncertain terms the path to optimal health through eating, moving and thinking right, and gives you the tools to make Big Changes. DO yourself a favour and read this book!

— ANDREW TAYLOR, AUTHOR, THE DIY SPUD FIT
CHALLENGE

No mater how long or how deeply you have suffered because of your weight, there is still hope. Read this book, embrace the Big Change methodology, and you will have your hope renewed.

— CHEF AJ, AUTHOR, THE SECRETS TO ULTIMATE WEIGHT LOSS

A wonderfully written book based in the science of nutrition and behavior, and is focused on not merely providing information, but truly empowering its readers to implement the life-changing habits.

— DEAN AND AYESHA SHERZAI, MDs, CO-AUTHORS, THE ALZHEIMER'S SOLUTION, CODIRECTORS OF THE BRAIN HEALTH AND ALZHEIMER'S PREVENTION PROGRAM AT LOMA LINDA UNIVERSITY MEDICAL CENTER

As one who struggled with and overcame a debilitating case of MS, I can relate to the inspirational wisdom and guidance of Josh and Howard. *Sick to Fit* is a step-by-step guide to turning one's life around by confronting excess weight and the accompanying physical challenges. But more importantly it brilliantly examines the necessary psychological foundation to be successful. This book is simplicity at its best, and it will leave the reader confident that anything is possible - if one is willing to devote the time, thought and energy. *Sick to Fit* is the definitive place to start!

— BOB CAFARO, AUTHOR, WHEN THE MUSIC STOPPED

Josh's story is extremely compelling and inspirational. His steps are clear and practical. His break with conventional thinking sharply contrasts him against ordinary weight loss books.

— Perry Marshall, CEO and Author of Ultimate Guide to Google AdWords and 80/20 Sales and Marketing and Evolution 2.0

Having undergone one of the most dramatic weight loss and fitness turnarounds you'll ever see, Josh LaJaunie is the mentor and coach who knows what needs to be done.

Anyone who is overweight or trapped in poor health can confidently follow the advice in Sick to Fit, knowing it's the blueprint for both Josh's own success, and the successes of the scores of people he has coached and inspired.

— Brian Wendel, founder and president of Forks Over Knives

A GIANT PROMISE THAT WILL MAKE
YOU WANT TO SMACK US

Y ou can lose a hundred or more pounds in the next 12 months and keep it off forever.

- Even if you're "genetically predisposed" to obesity.
- Even if you have the world's strongest sweet tooth.
- Even if you think you have no discipline, self-control, or willpower.
- Even if your weight has been yo-yoing since middle school, you've heroically taken up a new diet and pushed yourself at the gym until you reached your goal weight, only to see your progress all go down the drain as you let up or "celebrated" your way back to obesity.

And you can lose that weight permanently, more or less "by accident."

We know, this is such a huge claim, that you may want to smack us in the mouth right now. We get it. When I (Josh) weighed 420 pounds, I would have felt the same way.

Because by the time I maxed out at 420 pounds, and dealt with all the problems fat people deal with that skinny people can't even imagine (seat belt extenders, fear of restaurants with booth seating, breaking out in a sweat while trying to put on socks, industrial-sized tubs of Preparation H), I had been burned and disappointed so many times that I was sure every weight-loss technique and program in the world was utter and complete BS.

Previously, I had lost — and regained — 90 to 100 pounds at least three times. I knew all the diet hacks that worked, and I knew that none of them worked for long.

And when I was losing weight "successfully," it felt like a full-time job. Like all I could think about was the food I couldn't eat, and the couch I could have been sitting on while I was lifting weights.

If you had told me:

- that by making a modest set of changes in my life I could become a happy, vibrant, passionate, in-love-with-myself person...
- that as my transformation took place, I would naturally and effortlessly shed the 230 excess pounds I was carrying around...
- that living at my ideal weight was a hell of a lot more fun and pleasurable and rewarding than eating all my favorite foods...

I probably would have taken a swing at you.

"Don't get my hopes up!"

We don't expect to convince you that you can achieve the same outcome. So we're not asking you to believe us.

Instead, we're asking you to suspend your disbelief long enough to hear us out, and give our methods a try in your own life.

Your results are the only proof worth having, after all. Who cares whether someone else can lose weight, become an athlete, or stop trying to drown out his self-loathing with Little Debbie Nutty Bars, whiskey, and cocaine (as Josh did for years)?

We can stand up and say, "Look, this can be done."

We can offer you hope, a roadmap, a compass, and support along the way.

We can even introduce you to hundreds of other people who've made this same journey, and who generously credit us with being influential role models and guides.

But ultimately, you're the one who has to DO the thing.

We're not going to change your life — *you* are.

Howard is not going to chew the food at the end of your fork — *you* are.

Josh is not going to start walking around the block in your flip flops or running shoes — *you* are.

But don't worry, you've got us here to guide you, and to help make the journey just a tad less rocky than it was for us. And we believe in you. So if you believe in you, we are ready to begin!

The Good News

No matter where you are right now, you're in a really good place to begin your Big Change.

You know how we know that? Because you're here. You're reading this book.

Right now, you're motivated to get free from the pain, the shame, the guilt, the addiction, the embarrassment, and the discomfort.

You're fed up with what feels like a total lack of willpower and self-control.

You're tired of donning the "jolly" mask every day to put a brave face on your out-of-control existence.

Feel that energy. It's your purest and most powerful rocket fuel for this first stage of your Big Change journey.

You won't need it for long, as we'll see.

Which is a good thing, because we're willing to bet that your previous attempts to lose weight ended up crashing and burning because you ran out of that intense, high-octane motivation.

We won't let you make that mistake this time. We're going to toss the word "motivation" into the compost pile real soon. But for now, as long as it keeps you reading and starts you DOing, let's use those feelings of dissatisfaction and frustration for all they're worth.

Why Capitalize DO?

You may have already noticed that almost every time we use the word DO or DOing, it looks like our caps lock is stuck.

That's on purpose. Because the only thing separating those who succeed in losing weight and keeping it off, and those who never start, or yo-yo up and down, or lose a bunch of weight only to put it all back on as soon as the honeymoon is over, is that simple two-letter word: DO.

If you DO, you succeed.

As long as you pay attention to the results you get, and tweak your DOing until it gives you the results you want, you will get there.

Once you find your magic formula of the three big strategies you'll meet in this book — Menu, Movement, and Mindset — the fat will fall off.

You might be thinking: *What is it with you clowns? Another hyped-up claim?*

Not at all. Here's why:

That first thirty to one hundred pounds really doesn't want to be there. It may not feel like it, but you're actually working really hard to keep it on. Once you discover the principle of Naturally Attainable Quantities (NAQ) for the Human Animal (in Chapter 5), and you start working *with* your body instead of against it, you'll be shocked at how quickly you can drop inches off your waist and pounds on the scale.

We hope you're eager to dive in. Before you do, let's take a quick tour of where we're going, and why.

What's in This Book

In the next chapter, we're going to tell you the abbreviated version of our personal stories: how Josh went from 420 pounds to the cover of

Runner's World magazine, and Howard's less dramatic but still hugely gratifying change from unfit and unhappy chubby hubby to lean and joyful endurance athlete. We want to prove that you can apply these principles and methods and use them to change your life, no matter who you are or how dire or OK your current situation.

After that, we get into the Big Change methodology. We'll inoculate you against early-stage self-sabotage in Chapter 3. In Chapter 4, you'll get an overview of the three engines of Big Change. Chapter 5 covers the big idea that resolves all your confusion about diet: Naturally Attainable Quantities. We'll show you how this applies to food, and by extension to physical activity and beyond – and how filtering your questions and challenges through this one big idea simplifies the journey immensely. You won't need calorie charts or intricate training plans once you master the NAQ of living.

Armed with NAQ, you'll master the three big elements of Big Change: Menu, Movement, and Mindset.

In Chapter 6, you'll discover how and what to eat for rapid and effortless weight loss, and how to change tastes and habits to make your new way of eating your new default.

Chapter 7 will show you how to get moving, even if you're like Josh when he started, "jiggle jogging" at three miles an hour in the early mornings so no one would see him. And you'll learn how to gradually ramp up the intensity and duration until you see yourself — stay with us here — as an actual athlete.

Again, this may be the furthest thing from your mind right now, and you may be spluttering "BS!" as you read this, but we've seen it so many times it's just predictable to us now.

You're going to not only lose weight, but discover your biological essence, and we promise you it isn't "couch potato." Think about it: how could our species have survived if we couldn't have roused ourselves to vigorous activity when the need arose?

And — in arguably the most crucial part of the book (Chapter 8) — you'll discover the mental patterns and habits that fuel long-term success.

The thought patterns that turn weight loss into an afterthought rather than an obsession.

The beliefs that empower us to be truly happy with who we are, so we no longer have to constantly rely on the pleasure hits of junk food to boost our sagging morale.

And you'll discover how to cultivate those Mindsets in yourself.

In Chapter 9, we'll put it all together into a personalized plan that you can start following today to start seeing and feeling results tomorrow.

Before we dive in, though, we want to invite you to join us in the most important element for making and sustaining a change: community.

Think about it — didn't it take community to get you overweight and unhealthy?

- To supply you with unnatural quantities of hyper-delicious, hyper-fattening foods, and then pat you on the back as you consumed it?
- To make you feel bad about yourself, in subtle and not-so-subtle ways?
- If you're as obese as Josh was, to pigeonhole you into fat person roles, like "supportive best friend" or "life of the party"?

To break out of your unhealthy patterns, you need to find a new community.

People who will support you and challenge you.

People who care about you but don't buy your excuses because they recognize them from their own lives.

People who are five steps ahead of you, to encourage and inspire you, and people who are five steps behind you, to call forth your own greatness as you become a role model for others.

And people who will walk/run/jog/swim/bike next to you on your journey and become close allies and friends.

We've created such a community, which you can join on Facebook:

Facebook.com/groups/sicktofit

It's a closed group, which means we and our network of Big Change admins and alumni volunteers approve each and every member. This lets us keep it real and positive and evidence-based and helpful, and avoid the negativity that plagues too many online groups.

READER BONUSES

We want this book to be much more than just information; we want you to use it as a gym to strengthen your own Menu/Movement/Mindset muscles. Like a gym, we can give you the keycard and the towel and the water bottle, but you've got to lift the weights.

We've included lots of bonus material – think of it as your own personal trainer – to help you get the most out of the concepts and exercises in *Sick to Fit*. Audio and video interviews, Menu and Movement demonstrations, in-depth discussions of concepts we introduce here – all designed to help you DO sooner, better, and more sustainably.

You can access all these bonuses at SicktoFit.com.

The bonuses for this chapter are an audio and video about NAQ, and how the concept of Naturally Attainable Quantities can simplify your life and help you make good decisions.

Once you've joined and introduced yourself, it's time to get started on your own Big Change journey.

As your guides, let us introduce ourselves, and explain why you're in good hands.

2

WHY YOU MIGHT WANT TO LISTEN TO US

Josh's Story

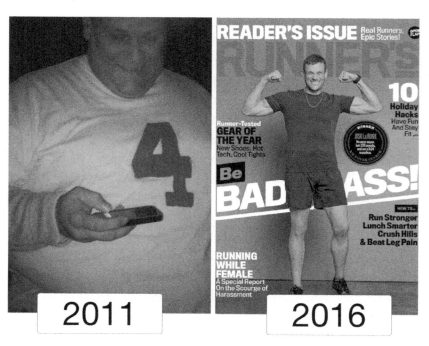

J osh LaJaunie here.

I am an unabashed Who Dat (Saints fan) with a last name that has Cajun South Louisiana written all over it.

I grew up on Bayou Lafourche in Thibodaux, Louisiana.

Growing up on the bayou has contributed to a lot of things in my life of which I'm immensely proud:

- My relationship with nature, which guides me now more than ever as I consider the right way to live a human life.
- The famous bayou "can-do, make-do" attitude and skill set, born from many trips to our hunting camp far from the nearest store, which allows us to transform an old rowboat, a roll of duct tape, and a can of Flex Seal into a Cajun submarine, and a sack of muddy potatoes into a delicious and filling *sauce patot* (potato stew).
- My love of music, Movement, and joyful communal celebration.
- The fierce love and loyalty of family.

My coonass (that's what some of us rural Cajuns proudly call ourselves) heritage also bred into me a relationship with food that was as intense as my love for family, nature, and music. We're famous for our food: our jambalayas, crawfish boils, étouffées (indescribably rich stews), beignets (deep-fried donuts), and of course our beloved po' boys (baguettes crammed with strips of the cheapest meat or fish you can find). I was in love with all of it, and ate it all the time, the more the better.

Even as I ballooned to north of 400 pounds. Even as I quit football, dropped out of college, started dealing drugs to pay for my growing cocaine habit — food was always my favorite pacifier, helping me ignore my values and ambitions along with my snowballing misery and shame.

Not that you could have picked me out of a crowd of my kin in those days. My bayou brothers and sisters are a hefty lot, celebrating our love of rich, sweet, salty, fatty, and highly processed foods three times a day, if not more.

My grandfather, Bam Bam, my role model in everything, weighed 380 pounds. My brother Dustin tipped the scales at 430 pounds. My mom and dad's combined weight was 700 pounds. If normal is what you see when you look around, then my morbidly obese 49.9 body mass index (BMI) was well within acceptable range. I was just a "good eater" in a culture where consumption is idolized, and every problem can be soothed with food.

Of course, I was never happy with my weight. Being a big guy may have been an asset on the high school football team, but it was always the quarterback and running backs who garnered the adoration of the girls. I tried to compensate by being the larger-than-life funny guy, the best friend, the guy who could score beer or weed, who could put together the wildest party, and who knew the best fishing spots and deer camps.

During my high school senior beach trip to Cancun, I was so self-conscious about my 300-pound body that I was a total stick in the mud. I wouldn't go to the beach or the pool. I told my friends that the trip was boring and no fun, which really pissed them off. Deep down, I was just ashamed to take my shirt off in front of them because I had recently discovered my first stretch marks.

I was always going on diets of one sort of another. I tried them all: Atkins, Paleo, Weight Watchers, Jenny Craig, high-protein, high-fat, fasting, powders, shakes, and pills. And they all worked great — for a little while.

I would lose 80, 90, even 100 pounds and reach whatever my latest magical target weight was.

Then, to celebrate, I would go right back to the foods and beverages that had made me fat in the first place — and in short order, gain back every single pound, plus some.

I didn't have a clue about what a *sustainable* way of eating was and I was completely ignorant of the science of nutrition, so I had no idea that certain diets simply cannot be maintained indefinitely, even if they are wicked effective at helping one shed excess weight at first.

The thing that worked the best for me, Xenadrine with Ephedra, was taken off the market by the FDA because the Ephedra was killing people. Cocaine worked too, but had other consequences that weren't so pleasant, like forcing me into becoming a dealer to afford it, along with cocaine's physical side effects (for me, these included rapid weight loss, dark circles under my eyes, and escalating paranoia).

I remember laying on a mattress, the sole piece of furniture in the townhouse I was renting with a bartending friend of mine. I didn't have the cash to repay my dealer, who had been known to shoot people for less. I didn't have money to pay the rent. I had stopped bartending and was just taking phone calls and selling coke. And as my financial situation deteriorated, I was consuming more and more of the coke myself.

After my mother gave me money to save my life and never asked questions or said a negative word to me; after a girl I loved died of a cocaine overdose (not dealt by me, but I had certainly contributed to her habit); after my beloved grandmother, my Memaw, died suddenly at the age of 67, something shifted in me and I knew I had a lot of making up to do. A lot of atoning and a lot of soul-searching.

I'll share more of my story — the happier parts — throughout this book. But what I want you to understand right now is that no matter how overweight you currently are, I get it.

I know the shame and the bravado, the frustration and hope, the desperation and despair. I know all the diet tricks. I know all the short-term hacks.

I know the physical discomforts: the chronic constipation, gut problems and their attendant terrible farts, hemorrhoids that made sitting or moving all but impossible, constant aches and pains, swelling, and smelly skin where I couldn't reach to wash.

And as you'll see, I discovered a way out. Three elements — Menu, Movement, and Mindset — that stacked on each other and created a foundation for radical change.

The change was slow at first, but gained momentum. I made tons of mistakes, and hundreds of wrong turns. One of the reasons for this book is to spare you as many of them as possible.

I'm still a work in progress. But now, unlike during those decades of obesity and self-loathing, I'm a happy work in progress.

And, in a curious mental shift, once all three elements were in place, weight loss became an afterthought, not the main goal. It's like I lost the last 120 pounds by accident, by focusing on making myself a better, more worthy, happier human being.

Oh, and just in case you're thinking, "Well, staying lean is easy for him. He's a professional athlete. He gets paid to run" — I've got news for you.

Aside from some free socks and half-price shoes, I don't get any compensation from running.

Instead, I make my money owning and running two businesses here in Thibodaux: a trailer park, and a private sewer company.

I spend long hours, day and night, troubleshooting and chasing down problems. I don hip waders and fish out used condoms and tampons and tube socks from pump impeller shafts. I repair broken motors and get covered in oil in 90 degree heat and 90% humidity. I settle fights among tenants, plug leaks, deal with constant storms and flooding, haggle with the Department of Environmental Quality — and much more.

I get up at 3 AM to run at 4, so I can start working by 6 or 7. I tell you all this not to brag, but to preemptively deprive you of some excuses why I can do it but you can't.

We all have shit to deal with in our lives. Mine has been pretty big and persistent (and literal, in my line of work), but probably you've got plenty of your own. Our struggles can either keep us down, or inspire us to greater heights. It's our choice — a concept I'll go into in depth in the Mindset section.

To watch videos of Josh's story, sign up for the free Reader Bonuses at SicktoFit.com.

For now, just know that my story hasn't been all butterfly kisses and unicorn farts.

Howard's Story

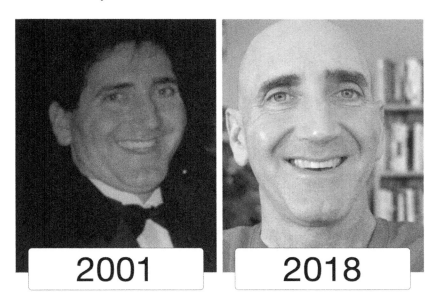

I was in pretty good shape when I met Josh LaJaunie, or so I thought.

I was a respected health educator, with two advanced degrees after my name.

I had co-written two important books on health and nutrition: *Whole*, by renowned researcher T. Colin Campbell, and *Proteinaholic*, by bariatric surgeon Garth Davis, MD.

I had a health consulting practice, in which I counseled and educated my clients on proper diet and exercise.

And I jogged sometimes, and played team sports, and did martial arts, and gardened. I was active and fit, I tell you!

Sure, I was maybe 25 pounds heavier than I had been in college, but that was no big deal. I just avoided horizontal stripes and made sure never to tuck in my shirt. The beach was out, too; I knew my dad bod was no advertisement for the services I was offering to others.

Sure, I was exhausted most of the time, and had trouble focusing on my work for more than an hour or two.

Sure, I avoided any sort of physical, mental, or emotional discomfort like the plague.

But – aside from my looks, my lack of energy, and my utter lack of courage – everything was fine.

Josh and I met through Facebook. Like thousands of others, I had seen Josh's before and after photos, and was astounded at the transformation. I thought that Josh would make a great guest on my Plant Yourself Podcast. So I messaged him to see if he'd be interested.

He was. In fact, it turned out that I was one of his heroes, because of my contributions to books that'd had such an influence on him.

We got chatting, and Josh sent me a document he'd written, about his background and struggles and transformation. He hadn't shown this to anyone before — not even his wife.

I read it and thought, "This story needs to be told." It was inspiring, it was instructive, and a lot of the advice was totally the opposite of what I'd heard and believed and taught in my own practice.

And it wasn't like my advice had turned me into a competitive runner, or even into a guy comfortable in swim trunks. All of my book learning and theory hadn't ever helped anyone the way Josh had helped himself.

I needed to know more.

We decided to write a book together. On a Monday in May, 2016, he drove up from the bayou to my home in North Carolina, and we worked together for five days.

Tuesday morning we went running. Our 6.8-mile run was barely a warmup for Josh, but was my longest effort in five years. Josh jogged beside me, coaxing me up tough hills as I stopped to walk and gasp and clutch my sides.

We returned to my house an hour later. Josh looked like he had strolled down to the mailbox and back; I looked and felt like I had crawled through mud and quicksand and semi-molten lava for a few thousand miles.

And here's what my idiotic brain was thinking: "Sure, Josh, it's easy for you. You don't know what it's like to have 20 extra pounds of fat around your middle as you try and run."

Luckily, I didn't blurt those words out. And I was truly mortified at having thought them. Really? The guy who used to weigh 420 pounds doesn't understand my middle-age chub? Give me a break.

The next day, I admitted to Josh that I'd had that thought. We both laughed. And I said that I wanted to run again the following morning. I would be tougher, and work harder so that Josh could get a challenging workout too.

Thursday morning, Josh was ready at 6 am. But the bastard was wearing a 20-pound weight vest.

Apparently he had brought it from Louisiana, as if he had anticipated my sorry-ass excuse and accordingly contrived a prop to blow it to smithereens.

This run was much worse. Josh ran ahead of me, and glanced back occasionally to confirm that I hadn't turned into a carcass in the reflected heat of the asphalt. But his goal here wasn't to coddle or encourage me; instead, it was to goad me to greater effort and grit and discomfort than I had voluntarily experienced in decades.

I finished that run with a short sprint to my mailbox. I was in agony. My core muscles were screaming. I could hardly breathe. My heart was jackhammering its way out of my chest.

And I was elated. Thrilled. Prouder than I had been of myself in years. And totally hooked on the idea of Better, the mantra that Josh had been reciting to himself throughout his own transformation, and was now sharing with anyone who cared to listen.

It was then that I realized: I wanted to share what Josh had figured out with the world, sure. I wanted to be more effective as a health educator and wellness consultant, absolutely.

But mostly I wanted it for myself. To partake of my own Big Change. To toughen myself up, so that I could withstand hard physical workouts — but also to toughen myself up emotionally, so that I could be more open and available and loving with others, rather than cocooning and staying cool and aloof so their suffering wouldn't trigger my own.

I wanted to be a man of my word, who kept his promises to himself and others. Who said no to junk food in private as well as in public. Who got up and exercised as long and as hard as he said he would, regardless of the desire to sleep in or take it easy, or put it off until tomorrow.

So on our last day together, Saturday, I told Josh that I was going to start training for a 50k race. He nodded warily (he'd heard that before), and showed me a website to search for nearby ultramarathons, and sent me a beginner's 50k training plan.

Now I would have to put in the work. To DO.

As I write this, I'm happy to report that with Josh's support and guidance every step of the way, I've put in that work.

I came in 20th in that 50k. Then I signed up for and ran a 10-miler, a half marathon, four marathons, two 10ks, and a 5k. The following year I ran that first 50k again, and came in 5th overall, 19 minutes faster than the previous race.

I'm lean. I'm fit. I can handle life's difficulties with a lot more resilience. And now that I walk my talk, I'm an infinitely more effective coach and teacher.

And a Cast of Thousands

Turns out I'm not alone in being inspired to make a Big Change by Josh.

Once Josh transformed his own body and mind and life, his family followed. Between them, his parents, his brother and sister, and his grandfather have lost a total of 900 pounds.

Friends and neighbors and customers and vendors also witnessed Josh's transformation from obese and unhappy to lean and vibrant. And many of them have adopted Josh's strategies for themselves, turning into healthy-eating athletes who embrace discomfort and challenge in their forever pursuit of Better.

The Missing Chins Run Club

When Josh got slightly famous, thanks to an appearance on the Rich Roll Podcast in December 2013, his sphere of influence grew to include hundreds of strangers who friended him on Facebook and Instagram.

Many of them were hundreds of pounds overweight, and had never met anyone who had overcome that particular challenge. With Josh as an example of what was possible with pragmatism and self-love, many of them doubled and redoubled their own efforts at Big Change.

In October 2016, Josh created a super-secret Facebook group after a conversation with a couple other ex-fat guys about needing some kind of virtual hangout to serve as a support hub and headquarters for all the obese and formerly obese guys who were at various stages of their own Big Change. The Missing Chins Run Club allowed members to vent, rant, bust balls, hold each other accountable, and connect deeply with each other and with their own awesome, heretofore-unimaginable, authentic human potential.

The Leadville Challenge

I met about a dozen of the Missing Chins in June 2017. Josh and some friends organized a pilgrimage to one of the most challenging races in the world: the Leadville Marathon and Heavy Half. The starting line elevation is just over 10,000 feet, while the highest point of the race, Mosquito Pass, tops out at just over 13,000.

The terrain is rocky, the winds are fierce, the sun is blazing, and the paths are steep and winding. The Heavy Half is about 15 miles, and the full marathon is the standard 26.2 miles with a total elevation gain of 6000 feet (meaning, as you're moving horizontally, you're also going up more than a mile). Some of us chose the heavy half, some the full.

And I was there to participate, as well as witness the courage and grit and preparation that allowed every single one of the Missing

Chins members who made the trip to Leadville, and to the finish line. It was an incredible privilege, to spend time among people who had overcome what most researchers believe is impossible and most people wouldn't even begin to attempt.

The Big Change Program

Meanwhile, Josh and I launched an online program to help more people lose massive amounts of weight, get fit, and rebuild their lives from the ground up. We dubbed it the Big Change Program.

The first Big Change Program launched in August 2016, and we felt confident enough to launch a second cohort in January 2017. Now we run them every couple of months.

By now, hundreds of people have participated, joining weekly online video meetings, journaling their daily progress and challenges in a forum, wrestling with a variety of homework assignments, and posting their workouts on Strava, a social media platform for athletes.

You'll meet some of those Big Changers in the bonus materials for this book, and get inspired by their remarkable stories of transformation. For now, here's the biggest takeaway from their experience (something we hear over and over in their forum posts): "I thought this was all about weight loss, but it's so much more."

The "more" differs from person to person, but a few things, we hear again and again:

- "For the first time I can remember, I really like myself, and I want to do kind things for my body."
- "I've gained control over my behavior, overcome binges and cravings, and I'm damn proud of myself."
- "I'm no longer a victim of my past."
- "I now push through discomfort to achieve my goals — I'm a real athlete. Me! I never would have believed it!"
- "I'm living my life as a healthy example to my family, friends, and coworkers. I've become a lighthouse, guiding others to health."

In fact, the unofficial tagline for the Big Changers, the way they frequently sign off their daily check-ins, is "Shine On!" Which Josh and I love, because that's how we can expand our own reach exponentially. And of course, we're all just ripples in that concentric circle of influence, with our own mentors and guides who empowered and anointed us to spread the message of Better.

To listen to some Big Changers talk about their own journeys, sign up for the free Reader Bonuses at SicktoFit.com.

By the third cohort, we were looking for a more robust online platform to host the Big Change Program. We knew of WellStart Health from a podcast interview I did with CEO Olivia Kelly, and when we asked her if we could try Big Change using her technology, she agreed.

This book comes out of our experiences guiding hundreds of people through Big Change: the Big Change Program and WellStart participants, as well as the hundreds of folks that Josh and I have worked with since the initial publication of Sick to Fit.

We've tried to take as much complexity as possible out of the journey. Because we've discovered that the simpler you make this whole change thing, the easier and faster you make progress.

We've also discovered that most people use complexity as a way of avoiding the DOing. This was my method for years: there was always another book to read, another gadget to buy, another room to repurpose, another trainer to see, before I could really get started and take action.

So here's where we do the big reality slap: If you want to use this book to change your life for the better, you're going to have to DO the work. Consistently. With as much commitment as you can muster.

You're going to have to be OK with discomfort. With cravings that you don't act on. With workouts that go on longer than you would like. With difficult conversations that convert your enablers into allies on your journey to Better.

We're not throwing you into the deep end, of course. We're big believers in small steps, gradual progress, and treating yourself with profound compassion and gentleness as you make this journey.

But we call BS on the common misuse of the phrase "progress not perfection" to excuse every lazy decision and justify every binge.

Beginning archers don't expect to hit the bullseye every time. But they still *try* to hit it every single time: they put great focus into each shot, and assess each miss to discover how to DO better next time. That's what we demand of ourselves, and ask of our students and clients.

If that sounds like more than you're willing to DO, we hope you'll reconsider. Because aiming for the bullseye is what's going to get you tangibly closer to where you want to be. Is it going to be easy? No. But it will be exciting, and it will be rewarding, if you are willing to DO the work.

Because the weight loss is not the point; it's an incidental byproduct of the true Big Change that happens when you retrain your brain to think like a healthy, confident human being. And that kind of change, a fundamental identity shift, takes work.

And man, it's so worth it!

Are you ready to take that first small step on the journey of a lifetime? If so, read on.

3

HOW TO PREVENT EARLY STAGE SELF-SABOTAGE

The heart of Big Change consists of three elements: Menu, Movement, and Mindset, which we'll cover in chapters 6-8. You'll discover the ideal human diet and how to approach it, the authentic human forms of Movement, and a Growth Mindset that turns your approach to health from frantic plate-spinning to your new normal.

But first, we need to deal with the ghosts of your prior failures to lose weight and get fit.

If you've never tried and failed before, we apologize for the insinuation. It's just that we — and everyone we know — have a ton of failures and disappointments and frustrations under our belts.

And if you approach Big Change with the same beliefs that you brought to your past efforts, you'll get the same results you've gotten before.

If you're like us, and like most of our clients, you're all too familiar with this scenario: you start some new diet or habit or routine with tons of motivation, DO really well for a time, and then hit a wall and give up.

When making a lifestyle change, you *will* have the inevitable challenges and setbacks; the philosophy you bring to that change will determine whether those challenges and setbacks are productive or just frustrating.

If they're productive, you'll gain momentum and continue, even when things get hard.

If all you get is frustrated, you'll give up.

So let's nip that pattern in the bud. Fortunately, it's really easy to do with the right philosophy of change.

Take your time with this chapter. As one of our star Big Changers, Sue Boyles, pointed out to us, "TELL THE READER THAT THIS IS SOME REALLY IMPORTANT SHIT RIGHT HERE."

Will do, Sue!

The Second Car in the Driveway

One morning several decades ago I (Howard) got up too early, skipped breakfast, and stumbled to my car to get to work on time.

I stepped on the brake, turned the key in the ignition, put the car in reverse, and eased off the brake — like I had done ten thousand times before.

But this time, I slammed to a halt after moving about three and a half feet. I was thrown back into my seat. I heard crunching. My heart began pounding like a heavy metal drummer.

Jolted into full wakefulness, I twisted around to see what had happened.

I had driven into my other car, which had been parked right behind the one I was driving out of my single-lane driveway.

I haven't engaged in that level of automotive cluelessness since that morning. But in other areas of my life, I can still be an expert at getting in my own way.

And I've noticed that my clients and students, too, often create predictable obstacles as they ramp up their own journeys to wellness.

In this chapter, we want to share three of the most common "second car in the driveway" Mindset mistakes — and provide some tips on navigating lifestyle and diet change so you don't crash before you even get moving.

Mistake #1: Insistence on Perfection

An old joke:

Henry is sitting on the porch next to his dog, Jake, who's howling like crazy.

Cloteal comes by and asks what's the matter.

"Oh, Jake's sittin' on a rusty nail," Henry says.

"Why don't he just get up?" Cloteal asks.

"'Cause it don't hurt enough yet."

Most of us have a lot of issues in our lives that simply "don't hurt enough yet." We may be annoyed at the extra 15 (or 115) pounds of fat on our frames, that broken bathroom fan, or our tendency to become belligerent with unhelpful call center reps — and we may complain and ruminate about these problems with regularity — but we generally just live with them rather than spending energy and other resources trying to solve them.

The problems rise to the level of "hurt enough yet" only when they tip past a threshold (like 300 pounds) or when an event (a house guest with really bad diarrhea) or outcome (not getting that incorrect $30 charge taken off your monthly cable bill) makes it clear that the status quo is no longer acceptable.

In other words, we delay taking action until it suddenly "hurts enough." That's when we feel the urgency of solving the problem. And then we want to solve it immediately, and completely, and forever.

In other words, we want to go from incompetence to perfection in a hot second.

In and of itself, aiming for perfection isn't a problem. In fact, it's usually admirable.

The problem comes when we make immediate perfection the only acceptable standard. When it comes to lifestyle and diet choices, we've been conditioned for years or decades to behave in certain ways. And all those factors are still very much in force when we muster the will to change.

Obstacles to success include:

- Our biological hardwiring to seek out super-rich foods and avoid strenuous exertion
- Our conditioned tastes and preferences
- Our immediate environments
- Our default systems for shopping, preparing food, relaxing after work, socializing, and entertaining
- Our social networks
- Our advertising-driven culture
- And many more...

Thinking that we can overcome all these obstacles to change in a single moment of intense motivation is an invitation to fail big-time.

We'll try to bite off more than we can chew. We'll split our focus between too many behavioral fronts, and fail to get lasting traction on any of them.

We'll exhaust ourselves and stress ourselves out, then return to the same unwanted behaviors we were trying to change. Because those behaviors allow us to self-soothe or self-medicate, or simply because we're too spent and exhausted to overcome our default habits.

So what are the ways to combat the initial impulse toward perfection?

1. Recognize the tendency

As I said, wanting to achieve perfection isn't the problem. It's when the pursuit of perfectionism causes us to overcommit and burn out that we get into trouble. So the first thing to do is to notice this tendency within yourself.

Does this pattern of overcommitting and burning out sound

familiar? In the past, have you gone "all-in" and then found your commitment wavering after a week or a month?

Have you bought all the gear and the clothes and rearranged your living room for the stationary bike or treadmill, put in an hour a day for a couple of weeks, and then found yourself only using it as an expensive drying rack two months later?

Have you thrown out all your junk food and filled your fridge with enough produce and herbal tonics to keep Gwyneth Paltrow in smoothies for a year, and then shamefacedly tossed the rotting veggies into the trash a week or two later because you didn't know how to prepare them?

Simply acknowledging that you have the tendency toward perfectionism is the first step. Realize that it comes from a good place. And remind yourself to cool your jets, and approach lifestyle change in a more sustainable way so that, this time, you can succeed.

2. Set mini-goals

Perfectionism thrives on a binary state of affairs: things are crap now, and they have to be marvelous. There's no in-between, no on-ramp, no pathway to success. It's "Beam me up, Scotty" or nothing.

Real life works differently. We make progress toward our goals in steps. This progress may be glacial or tectonic — small, almost imperceptible improvements, or bigger shifts — but rarely happens all at once.

So take advantage of the way reality works by identifying and working toward milestones along the way.

If your intention is to exercise hard for an hour a day, six days a week, and right now your fiercest exertion is operating the manual seat height adjustment on your minivan, then plan out a bunch of smaller goals along the way.

Maybe walk for 20 minutes three times a week. And then 22 minutes. Then 25. Then four times a week. Then five. And keep adding increments until you're where you want to be.

You get the idea. Break your ultimate goals into small steps (really, the smaller the better), and hold yourself accountable for achieving the possible rather than the unrealistically heroic.

3. Celebrate small wins

In addition to setting mini-goals, it's crucial to reward your brain by celebrating your progress.

The nice thing about having these mini-goals is that you get frequent positive reinforcement each time you reach one. In other words, ongoing motivation. So the lower you set the bar for each new achievement, the more small wins you experience, and the more frequent those boosts of motivation.

Think like a casino operator: you get people addicted to the slots not just by promising the extremely improbable gargantuan payout, but by giving them smaller wins along the way.

Instead of having your perfection-craving mind sabotage you by urging you to leap across a too-wide behavioral chasm, you can give it constant "we're on the right track" feedback to make it an ally in your transformation.

Mistake #2: Misinterpreting Failures

I would love to tell you that once you commit to a sustainable path of lifestyle improvement, you can simply stick to the plan and improve continually. That there won't be any backsliding, any doubts, any moments of weakness. That once you've sworn off certain foods and behaviors, you'll never look back.

But it just ain't so.

If you're human, then you will make mistakes.

The problem is not that you will make mistakes. The problem is not that you will experience failures along the way.

Mistakes and failures are perfectly natural, are to be expected, and frankly, they're the engines of your long-term success (I'll explain in a minute).

What will cause you to flame out is interpreting those mistakes and failures as signs that the whole project is doomed. Seeing mistakes as proof that you'll never succeed will kill your motivation to keep trying.

Let's say you decide to eliminate refined sugar from your diet. You've been perfect for a whole month, and then you're stuck in a deadly dull all-day sales meeting, complete with PowerPoint presentations and line graphs and spreadsheets, and you're seriously considering getting the insides of your eyelids tattooed with images of your favorite Marvel superhero — when someone arrives with a box of Krispy Kreme assorted.

Your willpower shot, you succumb to peer pressure and have just one bite of a cruller . . . which leads to another bite and another, and then to – what the hell! – a cinnamon dusted and a raspberry-filled chocolate glazed.

Later that night, you think back on the carnage and decide that you simply don't have what it takes to give up sugar. Rather than resuming your avoidance of sugar right after the binge, you give up altogether and add cookies, donuts, and sodas back into your diet on a regular basis.

Here are three antidotes to the despair that comes from giving too much power to your inevitable failures.

1. Reinterpret failures as fight-thrus

In their wonderful book *Organize Tomorrow Today*, Jason Selk and Tom Bartow describe the three stages of successful habit change:

1. **Honeymoon:** You're just starting, you're totally psyched, motivated, and energized; everything seems easy and hunky-dory.
2. **Fight-thru:** You're stressed, in a challenging situation, exhausted and emotionally strung out, and are sorely tempted to fall back on your old default patterns rather than put the extra energy into maintaining your new habit.

3. **Second nature:** You can maintain your new habit no
   matter what life throws at you.

The second phase, "fight-thru," is the key to success on your habit-change journey. The trick to winning fight-thrus is to target a habit or behavior that you can achieve roughly four times out of five.

That's right: your goal here is to earn a perfect B minus: 80 percent.

If you lose every single fight-thru, then you've set your sights too high at this point in time. You've fallen into the perfectionist trap, and so are likely to end up making zero (or perhaps even negative) progress. Find a smaller step you can take, and chalk up those wins while building up your fight-thru muscle.

If you win every single fight-thru, then you're probably not making real progress either. You're in a holding pattern, not challenging yourself to achieve meaningful changes, which require more effort. Now is the time to go after a slightly bigger accomplishment.

But if you win four out of five fight-thrus, then you're in the sweet spot. You know that you've chosen a worthy goal, because it challenges your current capability by just a bit, and you get positive reinforcement every time you succeed.

The key is not to beat yourself up for that one-in-five failure, but instead to interpret it as the event that moves you forward.

Instead of dreading and avoiding situations where you might fail, you can then look forward to them. Failing and picking yourself up isn't a detour on the road to success; it's the only way you can make progress.

That is, *if* you know how to prepare for and learn from those failures. Which brings me to the other two antidotes.

2. Anticipate fight-thrus

It's one thing to fail from time to time. It's another to be constantly surprised by that failure, to the point where you keep falling into the same trap time after time.

Remember, you're not *trying* to fail one time out of five, or giving yourself an advance pass to do so. It's just what happens when you've picked an appropriately challenging goal.

As you approach each situation, don't just whistle a happy tune and hope for the best. Instead, anticipate and plan for those situations where you're most likely to lose a fight-thru. Perform what decision scientist Gary Klein calls a "pre-mortem." Picture the impending fight-thru in your mind. Play out the scenario and give it two endings: defeat and victory.

Start with defeat. Imagine yourself failing spectacularly, noticing the moves you make (and fail to make).

Pay attention to how you set yourself up for failure (for example, by saying to yourself something like, "I wonder if I'll be strong enough to resist those donuts").

Notice how your tension dissolves once you give in and take the first bite. And then notice how you think to yourself, "Oh, what the hell, I might as well finish it."

Then observe how shame drives you to eat a second, and then a third donut.

Next, replay the scene but give it a happy ending. What has to happen differently for that happy ending to feel realistic?

Do you counter that initial doubt with a strong reminder of your aspirational identity or big goals?

"I don't eat that stuff. It's not food for me. There's no need to wonder if I can resist, because eating that is simply not in the realm of possibility."

When the box of donuts passes in front of you, do you have a response ready that makes your decision clear without causing conflict or unpleasantness?

"No thanks, my doctor wants me to stay away from desserts for a while."

And if you do end up taking a bite, what's your damage control strategy?

"Whoops, I lost focus for a second there. Now I'm going to count to 20, remind myself of my big goals and why they're important to me, and quietly put the rest of the donut in the trash can. I don't have to lose control and go into a full-on binge just because I made one tiny mistake."

By engaging in "prospective hindsight" (a fancy way of saying, "Imagine that the future has already happened"), you can use those high-risk-of-failure situations to increase your skills and get closer and closer to the behaviors and habits you aspire to. When you imagine success vividly, focusing on your thoughts and behaviors, you build the same brain pathways that form in response to actual experience.

3. Learn from failures

Let's say the pre-mortem didn't lead to success in a fight-thru – or that a failure snuck up on you. The next step is to debrief what happened, so you can do better next time.

Here we recommend leadership development expert Peter Bregman's FAST Assessment, in which you ask and answer the following questions:

- What was I **Feeling**? (emotions)
- How was I **Acting**? (actions)
- What was I **Sensing** in my body? (physical sensations)
- What was I **Thinking**? (thoughts)

The data you glean from an honest, non-dramatic FAST Assessment will help you succeed next time in a similar or even more challenging situation. At the very least, you'll know one more thing *not* to do. Recalling how you reacted in these four domains is fodder for more accurate and relevant pre-mortems; it will allow you to prepare better for future fight-thrus. (We'll cover this methodology in depth in the next chapter.)

Reader Bonus

To eavesdrop on a coaching session that includes a FAST Assessment, sign up for the free Reader Bonuses at SicktoFit.com.

Mistake #3: Misinterpreting Successes

To recap: aiming too high can lead to catastrophic failure, and getting emotionally battered by our inevitable failures, whether caused by overreaching or simply because we're human, can lead to giving up. The third way we sabotage our success is by getting overconfident when we do have some early successes.

As we learned from Selk and Bartow in *Organize Tomorrow Today,* the first phase of habit change is usually the honeymoon. Everything goes great at first. As a result, we can get lulled into a false sense of security and let our guard down.

As The Grateful Dead sang in "Uncle John's Band": "When life looks like easy street, there is danger at your door."

It's helpful to better understand why behavior change can be so easy at the beginning. According to behavioral scientist BJ Fogg's Behavior Model, we can predict behavior almost algebraically:

$$\text{BEHAVIOR} = \text{MOTIVATION} + \text{ABILITY} + \text{PROMPT}$$

Let's forget about the prompt for now and just focus on motivation and ability. Basically, we will do a behavior if we want to do it (motivation) and we can do it (ability).

That's pretty obvious.

What's less obvious is that there's a tradeoff between the two: as motivation increases, the more likely it is that we'll do difficult things. And as our ability to perform a behavior increases, we need less motivation to do so.

An extreme example is lifting a car to save your child. It's really hard, but you're highly motivated to do it. But there are plenty of everyday examples as well — like when you find out that you are pre-diabetic and so you finally manage to eat healthier because you're scared of developing the full-blown disease.

The problem is that the initial flood of motivation tends not to last. It's fine for short-term heroics (like lifting cars). It works less well for long-term behavioral change. Once we get past the honeymoon period, motivation is extremely fickle. We can't will ourselves to be motivated. We can't choose our motivation level at any given moment.

I might be very motivated right now to get up tomorrow and go to the gym, but I can't bottle that motivation and drink it at 5:30 AM, when all I want to do is clutch my pillow and keep my eyes closed against the coming day.

So we have to accept reality: that our motivation will wane. And that when it does, new behaviors that require us to stretch our ability will be harder to maintain. Initial success is absolutely no guarantee of sustainable success. We cannot be complacent when the first days or weeks turn out really well.

Here are three tactics for interpreting early success in the most empowering long-term way.

1. Be happy

The good news is, you've achieved initial success. This means that you've chosen something that's actually possible.

To use a ridiculous example: if your desired behavior was flight (à la Superman, not Chuck Yeager), then you wouldn't succeed even once, even with infinite motivation.

So early success confirms that you've chosen a behavior you have the ability to perform, even if you won't be able to do it every single time in every single circumstance.

2. Be wary

Don't get complacent. Celebrate your successes, but simultaneously recognize that your desired behaviors will feel harder as your motivation wanes and other life stressors assert themselves.

Keep looking forward for challenging moments. Keep scanning the horizon for potential fight-thrus. And do pre-mortems in which you take into account how you will feel when the initial flush of motivation has worn off.

3. Spend motivation to increase ability and add prompts

Remember BJ Fogg's formula:

$$\text{BEHAVIOR} = \text{MOTIVATION} + \text{ABILITY} + \text{PROMPT}$$

Because motivation and ability work together in a see-saw fashion to predict behavior, when motivation to do a thing is high, our ability can be low (not zero, but low) and we'll still do it.

The same is true in the other direction: when our ability is high (i.e., the behavior is easy for us), we require very little (but not zero) motivation.

For example, most of us are quite good at brushing our teeth. We keep a toothbrush and tube of toothpaste in the bathroom, and know exactly how to perform the act. So even when we're tired and just want to fall into bed (low motivation), we still brush our teeth every single night.

Here's the ninja move regarding early successes: use them to render future motivation unnecessary. Motivation is already running high during the honeymoon phase. Early success increases that motivation, which in turn can support further wins, in a positive feedback loop.

But you know that motivation wanes. So spend it now to increase your ability, which is a much more stable quality.

For example, if you're motivated to eat right because of a health scare or invitation to a beach party or summer wedding, spend some of that motivation increasing your long-term ability to eat right.

You might take a healthy cooking class, or watch some videos and emulate the recipes, or ask a wellness coach to give you a healthy food tour of your local supermarket.

Or you might spend some of that motivation on upgrading your kitchen, increasing your ability to cook healthy meals by giving yourself enjoyable tools that encourage your desired behaviors.

You can also use some of your motivation during the honeymoon phase to optimize the third variable on the right side of Fogg's equation: the prompt.

Optimize the Positive Prompts in Your Environment

A prompt is a reminder or cue that exists in your environment that you respond to in a predictable way.

Most of us are familiar with the negative prompts in our lives — the office clock striking three that sends us to the vending machines, the Little Debbie end cap display at the Piggly Wiggly, the dessert menu at The Cheesecake Factory.

But there are positive prompts as well — and you can intentionally engineer them to support your desired behaviors. By keeping the floss next to your toothbrush, you make it easier to remember to floss. The act of brushing triggers the impulse to floss.

During the honeymoon phase, set up new prompts, and increase the visibility and intensity of existing ones.

For example, you can stock your fridge with baby carrots, celery, cherry tomatoes, oil-free hummus, salsa, and fresh berries, so you have new go-to snacks when you get the munchies.

You can put that wedding invitation on your fridge door so you remind yourself of your reason for making a change every time you open it.

You can buy a fitness tracker or glass water bottle to serve as a visual cue reminding you to walk or hydrate. (My prompt to drink more water is a half-gallon Mason jar on my desk. When it's full, I drink. When it's empty, I refill it.)

You can register for a local 5k race and put the event in your calendar.

If you're proactive about spending early stage motivation, you'll be more likely to continue on a path of progress even when that motivation inevitably wanes, because you've enhanced Ability and installed and intensified Prompts.

Ready for the Journey

The purpose of this chapter was to give you some tools to avoid the most common forms of self-sabotage that accompany the early stages of the Big Change journey.

Our hope is that, armed with awareness, you can avoid these Mindset obstacles entirely, or at least recover from them quickly, without having undone a lot of progress toward your goals.

It's like being awake enough to swerve and avoid that second car.

Or, even better, getting in that second car and pulling straight out onto the road to success.

Now it's time to build the engine – three engines, actually – that will propel you forward.

4

THREE ENGINES OF CHANGE

N ow that we know how to avoid the early pitfalls, let's fire up the three engines of positive lifestyle change: the big ideas that we will return to again and again as we pursue our ideal weight, our fitness goals, and our best, most authentic, happiest selves.

Josh here. As I said already, I had lost significant amounts of weight multiple times before I was able to crack the code and make that weight loss sustainable. Now, losing a hundred pounds is no small feat, so clearly I was doing a bunch of things right even in those early attempts. I was eating better (although far from optimally, and miles from sustainably) and I was moving more (although through a limited range and variety of exercises).

But I hadn't yet figured out any of the Mindset stuff that turned the project from one of losing pounds as quickly and painlessly as possible into whole-life improvement. I also hadn't mastered the three engines of change: really simple rules that, if we follow them, guarantee success.

Engine #1: Results Dictate Sufficiency

In this culture, losing weight and getting fit can be incredibly confusing. It's hard to know who to believe. Just look at all the different diets out there: low carb, Atkins, low fat, keto, Hollywood Cookie, paleo, Whole30, raw, vegetarian, and on and on.

And once we choose one, how strict do we have to be? 24/7 without deviation? A cheat meal here or there? Exceptions for special occasions?

And how much food should we eat? If you're as overweight as I was, you probably have the ability to stuff yourself far past the point of satisfied, full, or even comfortable.

Exercise can be even more complicated: Which exercises? How many sets? How many reps per set? How much weight? How often?

I used to drive myself crazy with these questions. I was always second-guessing myself, always doubting my choices, and always vulnerable to the latest article, diet book, friend's pronouncement, or fitness guru's system.

So I would lurch from protocol to protocol, exhausting myself and never giving anything a chance to prove itself and really work.

Then one day it dawned on me that I could make things a hell of a lot easier, by applying one simple rule:

RESULTS DICTATE SUFFICIENCY

This was the rule I had been using for years to run my businesses.

If I was fixing a broken sewer pump, how did I know whether I had succeeded? It had nothing to do with how many hours I had put into the repair, or how many calories I'd burned, or how much I'd spent on parts at Lowes. The only thing that mattered was whether the pump was working properly again.

If the results were what I wanted, then the effort and other inputs were sufficient.

If the pump still didn't remove waste water, or didn't do it fast enough, then it didn't matter how hard I sweated or how much money I charged on my business credit card. My inputs were insufficient for the task at hand.

At Sick to Fit, we all but worship results. Not necessarily for their own sake, but because they are the only valid feedback we have on what we're doing.

The Scale

Most dieters have a complicated relationship with the bathroom scale.

We want to know that we've lost weight, but we can get really depressed if the needle moves in the wrong direction.

We know that our weight can fluctuate day to day for lots of reasons having nothing to do with our dieting success (like our hydration level, constipation, more or less glycogen in the liver, and for many ladies, that time of the month), and yet we can still freak out if we've gained a pound from one day to the next.

We can also get addicted to the scale's feedback, to the point where we can check obsessively, and hang our entire self-worth on that one number.

None of that is helpful.

But it's also not a great idea to get rid of our scale and just fly blind. As Glenn Livingston points out in *Never Binge Again*, a pilot flying from New York to London wouldn't throw away their navigation instruments just because they veered off course a couple of times.

And an automobile driver would never tape over their speedometer because "my driving speed doesn't define me as a person."

So step on your scale daily, and record your weight. But instead of relying on that day's number to gauge your progress, I recommend using a 21-day running average (Dan Ariely's smart scale, available at shapa.me, does this for you automatically) so that random and day-to-day fluctuations don't confuse or demotivate you.

If your weight is moving in the right direction at a speed you're happy with, then you know your weight-loss efforts are sufficient. If it isn't, then something needs to change.

If you've plateaued far above your ideal weight, or see the scale moving in the opposite direction, it doesn't matter how compliant you've been with your diet or workout regimen. It's time to DO different. DO more. DO better.

If I had stuck to what got me from 420 pounds to 320 pounds, I would have never made it to 200 pounds. Plateaus are overcome by pragmatism and an orientation towards progress. Sounds simple, but it took me a while to figure it out.

Let Results Dictate Sufficiency.

Performance

Of course, your weight on the scale isn't the only measure worth taking and paying attention to.

It's great if the sewer pumps I own work well, but if my business isn't earning sufficient profit to support me and my family, then I need to change something—and keep making changes until the situation improves. This may mean outsourcing maintenance, or requesting a rate hike, or making deals to increase my customer base.

When I started tracking my workouts and caught the DO Better bug, I set performance goals for myself. Run a mile in under 18 minutes. Then 15, then 12, then 10.

Now I can run a mile in 5 minutes and 39 seconds. And I got there by hard training, sure, but also through smart and effective training. I let the results I was achieving determine the sufficiency and correctness of my training and dietary choices.

You don't have to start competing in races to track your performance. If you're walking, jogging, or running, get a GPS-enabled watch or download a Movement tracking app like Strava or MapMyRun to your smartphone. Or just mark out a mile route and see how long it takes you to DO that mile each day.

Business strategist Peter Drucker wrote that what gets measured, gets managed. It's true in business, and it's true in our everyday lives.

Subjective Measures

Of course, not every outcome can be turned into a number.

We don't want to live in a world where the only things that are valued are the ones that can be measured. What about happiness, passion, curiosity, wonder, and love? Whatever qualities or experiences you want in your life, you need to pay attention to them and whether you're getting them in sufficient quantity, frequency, and intensity.

Do you want to be a happy person? Most of us do. Your Menu, Movement, and Mindset choices will have a huge influence on your happiness. If you aren't as happy as you'd like, then you may have work to do in one or more of those areas.

Try something. Maybe start a meditation practice. Maybe replace a boring gym class with an energetic dance class. Maybe start the day with two cups of water before you start eating. And see what that does to your mood.

Use your progress toward your goals to inform your day-to-day actions and decisions, and your results will become a powerful engine of transformation.

Engine #2: Turn a Bad Day into Good Data

It's easy to say that Results Dictate Sufficiency, but what do we do when our results suck?

When we go off the rails and binge on some junk food we swore we'd never eat again?

When we sleep in and hit snooze a dozen times and totally blow off our planned workout?

I (Josh) have been there so many times, and for years I would totally beat myself up over the screw-ups.

I'd talk to myself like this:

"You fricking loser. You have no willpower. You're weak and pathetic. You suck. No wonder you're such a fat, ugly piece of..."

The Shame Game

You might think that verbally assaulting myself was a brave thing to do — that by acknowledging my failure and making it hurt, I'd do better next time.

But that's not how it went.

Paradoxically, that kind of self-shaming actually let me off the hook. Like somehow I had "paid" for my failure by taking this kind of abuse.

What I eventually discovered was that shaming myself wasn't brave, and it certainly wasn't effective. Instead, it was a copout that allowed me to avoid responsibility for my food lapses and blown-off workouts — for the lousy results I was getting.

Not only that, my negative self-talk pretty much doomed me to continued failure. It insisted that my messing up was:

- **Pervasive**, not specific: I hadn't made a poor choice; I was a totally awful human being.
- **Permanent**, not temporary: I hadn't just slipped up once or twice; my entire life was a giant screw-up.
- **Personal**, not situational: I was the source and the cause of all my problems, and therefore could never escape them.

So rather than being an impassioned call for bettering myself, my self-loathing self-talk was a voodoo-like curse that made me not even want to keep trying.

While it can feel, at the time, like we're being "responsible" by making ourselves suffer mentally and emotionally for our sins, the truth is, we automatically suffer when we make a bad choice — in our weight, our health, our well-being. Adding an additional layer of shame doesn't in any way increase our motivation or ability to DO better next time.

Instead, it signals that we really are NOT responsible for our outcomes, by globalizing our unworthiness and inability to change.

Wallowing in shame is much easier than doing the hard work of actually getting better.

After all, what's the point in putting in the effort when you're bound to fail?

It's Just Data

Eventually I figured out (and plenty of research backs this up) that our screw-ups and bad choices are valuable to us only to the extent that we can learn from them, and DO better next time.

In order to cultivate this skill of "turning a bad day into good data" — to borrow a phrase from a great book, *Change Anything* — we have to turn that shame-based perspective on its head.

Rather than predicting future failures, our poor choices become just that — poor choices. Good people make bad decisions sometimes, and we can make bad decisions and still be basically good and worthy and competent. Those lapses are temporary, and we can regain control and mastery over our actions and words. And our internal good qualities are more than a match for external temptations, even if sometimes we need to do some work to strengthen our ability to combat those temptations.

Curiosity

Instead of coming at ourselves with the shiv of judgment, let's look at past lapses through the kaleidoscope of curiosity.

Curiosity is one of the coolest and most productive of all emotions. For one thing, being curious is pleasurable, like happiness or joy, so when we experience curiosity, we like how it feels. Being curious isn't something we have to force ourselves to do.

Second, curiosity is different from the other positive emotions in that it's always within easy reach.

What I mean by that is, to feel the other positive emotions we typically require that life be a certain way: in order to be happy, or joyful, or peaceful, we have to have experiences that make us happy or joyful or peaceful. It's hard to be elated if I'm stuck on bumper-to-bumper traffic on the 405 and I'm late for a sales call and my small intestines feel like I ate deep-fried shrapnel for breakfast.

But I can instantly become curious about all of those experiences just by making the decision to be curious about them. Where do I feel the stress of the traffic jam in my body? What is my heart doing right now as I imagine my boss yelling at me for blowing the deal? What does deepening my breath do for the churning in my gut?

Third, curiosity is one of those emotions that automatically shifts how we use our brains. To be curious means to pay attention in an open and non-judgmental way (because judgment is the opposite of curiosity, as it insists, "I totally understand this now, and here's how it is, and so there's no need to be curious about it anymore").

The part of our brain that handles curiosity, the prefrontal cortex, is also the part that does long-term thinking, planning, rational decision–making, and strategic inhibition of impulsive behavior. When the prefrontal cortex lights up, it dims the fear center — the fight-or-flight region of the brain that interprets traffic and tardiness as dangerous predators and floods our body with chemicals that motivate us to "kill or run away."

When we activate the prefrontal cortex through curiosity, we move out of fight-or-flight. We can regain our perspective and our ability to be creative, so that we can weigh options and figure out how to do better, starting NOW.

How to Cultivate Curiosity

The thing about curiosity is that while it's always a choice, for most of us it's not a habit. So if we want to automatically get curious, rather than judgmental, when we stumble or make bad choices, then we have to train ourselves to be curious under less stressful circumstances so that curiosity is available to us when we need it most.

It's like shooting a thousand layups a day by yourself so you can hit one in the fourth quarter of a real basketball game.

Psychiatrist Judson Brewer, in *The Craving Mind*, a wonderful book about using mindfulness to overcome addiction, shows that meditation is one of the most effective ways to practice curiosity on a daily basis. By sitting down and consciously turning the kaleidoscope of curiosity on our bodies and breath and sensations and thoughts, and bringing our focus back again and again as we get distracted, we can build a "curiosity circuit" in our brains that makes it easier to trigger curiosity even in the face of discomfort and other negative emotions.

We'll cover meditation — and its importance in your Big Change journey — later in this book. For now, let's talk about how to use curiosity once we have it in our toolbox.

Post-Mortem and Pre-Mortem

In the last chapter, we encountered the principle of getting curious about failure so we can learn from it. These two techniques, the post-mortem and the pre-mortem, are the main cylinders of that "turn a bad day into good data" engine. Together, they provide the power and torque required for us to learn from our past mistakes and win our future fight-thrus.

The post-mortem enables us to learn from our experiences.

Instead of beating ourselves up and seeing past mistakes as proof of our immutable weak character, we focus clearly on a single point in time when we were weak, or confused, or in over our head — on that one decision that led to poor choices rather than good ones.

And we do all that without shame, which as we've seen only reinforces our helplessness.

Here's how to do the post-mortem once you've had a binge or other suboptimal experience.

Post-Mortem Instructions

1. Cut through any shame about your behavior.

If you find yourself overwhelmed by shame, guilt, worry, and disappointment, don't compound it by feeling ashamed of being ashamed. That's a hall-of-mirrors mind trick you want to avoid.

Instead, get curious about shame itself: What does it feel like in the body? Where is it most intense? What color is it? Temperature? Texture? How does it move? What does it weigh? Does it shift under the gentle scrutiny of your curiosity?

You'll find that with practice, curiosity weakens shame, and allows you to move past it without resistance or avoidance.

2. Re-experience the scene.

Don't just think about the situation where you made a choice you wish you hadn't, but really put yourself back in it. Use all your senses. What are you seeing? Hearing? Smelling? Feeling?

Go deep here, like you're wearing a vintage circa-2025 Virtual Reality headset. Really bring yourself back into the scene. Watch it play out. Watch yourself move through the situation from start to finish.

If you feel shame bubble up as you do this, return to step one and just get curious about the shame. It will subside.

3. Identify the critical moment.

The "critical moment," in the language of *Change Anything*, is that point at which you first took an action or believed a thought that led to the undesired outcome.

Maybe it was when you decided to eat a single Dorito at the buffet.

Or when you believed the little voice in your head that said, "This is a special occasion — we can break our rules for once."

Or when the alarm went off and you hit snooze instead of getting out of bed and putting on your workout gear.

4. Do the FAST Assessment.

The FAST Assessment, as we saw in the previous chapter, is all about identifying your contribution to the situation.

At that critical moment, what were you Feeling? How did you Act? What were you Sensing? What were you Thinking?

Get very specific here. The goal is to pinpoint where you could have done one thing differently to achieve an entirely different outcome.

5. Brainstorm other choices in that moment.

Now play with other options for yourself in that moment. And "play" is the operative word here. Be playful — it increases your creativity, counteracts shame, and makes it far more likely that you'll recall your insights and decisions in the future when you really need them.

Don't just brainstorm "rational" choices. Come up with fun stuff. For that single Dorito, you might come up with the following:

- Instead of eating the Dorito in my hand, I throw it like a ninja star and embed it in the wall.
- Before I reach for the Dorito, I drop and DO 20 pushups.
- Before I come to the party, I eat a large salad with a baked potato smothered in salsa and sautéed onion and mushroom so I'm totally not tempted by a fricking Dorito.

Note that in that last choice, the critical moment turned out to be well before the moment of indiscretion. You'll find this a lot — the real turning point, the "root cause" of your behavior, occurred well before the "symptom" that looked like the poor choice. When that happens, simply perform a new FAST Assessment on the newly discovered critical moment when you left home while you were still hungry.

6. Reshoot the scene with a happy ending.

After you've gone through a bunch of options (at least three, but the sky's the limit), rewrite the scene. Then run it in your imagination, aiming for as an immersive experience as before.

See what you see. Feel what you feel. Hear what you hear. Smell what you smell. Even though it's an imaginary future, do your best to experience it as if it's happening right now.

And watch yourself sense, feel, think, and act your way to a positive outcome.

7. Codify your choice with a When–Then plan.

Once you've identified a plan of action that would have worked in that situation, codify it so you have access to it in the future — which is the point of this whole exercise.

Psychologist Robert Cialdini, in his book *Pre-Suasion*, refers to this progress of codification as an "if/when-then plan."

As in, "**If** I know I'm going to a party where I'll be tempted to eat something I don't want to, **Then** I will have a healthy meal ahead of time."

Or, "**When** I see a bowl of Doritos, **Then** I will take three deep breaths and find a glass of water to drink instead."

From Crash and Burn to Minor Incident

As you first practice the post-mortem, you'll be focusing on the big disasters: bingeing on an entire box of Mint Milanos, having four alcoholic beverages to "take the edge off" one evening, or blowing off your morning walk to stay in bed and scroll through Instagram on your phone.

But as you get more experienced and catch and correct your behavior before going off the deep end, you'll start to apply the post-mortem technique to thoughts and behaviors that are less and less of a "big deal."

Business consultant Matthew Syed calls this approach "Black Box Thinking," in his book of the same name. Whenever a plane crashes, the aeronautics industry pores over the data captured in its recovered black box so they can learn from the failures and prevent them from happening again. Thanks to that consistency and commitment, flight has become safer and safer over time.

But they don't just wait for disasters in order to learn, Syed reminds us. Whenever a light malfunctions, or landing gear gets stuck for a moment, or there's a near-miss, aviation experts still perform a full post-mortem so that these not-disasters, too, can contribute to the industry's wisdom and improved performance over time.

Eventually, through diligent practice, as post-morteming becomes second-nature to you, your mistakes and failures will become less and less significant.

Pre-Mortem Instructions

The pre-mortem is the same as the post-mortem, except that you're applying the technique to the future.

Once you've accumulated a library of post-mortems, you'll be able to predict with a lot of confidence when you'll likely to face a critical moment in the future.

"I've messed up at potlucks in the past. There's one coming on Thursday at the kids' school, and I'd better come up with a strategy to stick to my diet."

"I've got a late call next Monday night, and a 5:30am spin class on Tuesday morning that I'm in danger of blowing off. I need to figure out how to get enough sleep so I can make that class, or else find a different workout later in the day."

"The whole family is coming over for Thanksgiving, and they're used to me cooking all the foods I don't eat anymore. I'd better make a plan or else I'll end up gaining 20 pounds and feeling lousy."

Once you've identified the critical moment, run the post-mortem technique in your imagination.

Start by seeing yourself making a decision you'll regret:

Watch yourself eat three heaping plates of pasta salad and buffalo wings dripping with ranch dressing at the potluck.

See yourself slamming the snooze button six times, missing spin class, and spending the entire day in a sluggish fog.

Play the movie of you cooking — and pigging out on — turkey, pecan pie, sweet potatoes dripping with butter, and more. And then laying on the couch in a swirling stupor of tryptophan, queasiness, and regret while the Lions and the Bears battle it out on TV.

Then apply the rest of the post-mortem steps and watch yourself succeed gloriously, whatever that looks like to you.

Your "when-then plan" is your new best friend, your anchor, as you prepare for the upcoming critical moment.

If it goes according to plan, awesome. If not, you know what to do, right? A post-mortem. Wash, rinse, and repeat.

Engine #3: Make Decisions Once

There's a lot of chatter these days about willpower being a limited resource. Meaning, if you resist eating a chocolate chip cookie in the morning, you're more likely to cheat on your spouse in the afternoon. If you bite your tongue during a meeting at work and don't call your idiotic coworker an idiot, you're more likely to pig out later.

Even if you don't have to exercise willpower to resist some temptation, this theory says, the very act of making repeated decisions can fatigue willpower. Plan a wedding reception or decorate a bedroom now, and you're more likely to cuddle up with a full pint of Cherry Garcia later.

And the media are full of stories on how overachievers like Mark Zuckerberg and Barack Obama intentionally limit the number of decisions they make daily by always wearing the same outfit and eating the same breakfast.

Researchers like Roy Baumeister, coauthor of *Willpower*, and others have even come up with fancy social science names for this phenomenon: decision fatigue, and ego depletion.

Now, we have our doubts about all this research. New studies aren't replicating the results of the earlier ones (check out this Slate.com article from 2016 if you want to geek out on the topic: http:// j.mp/ego-depletion), and many of the types of things people did in those original studies (like stick their hands in ice water) aren't really relevant to everyday life and our actual goals and desires.

It does make intuitive sense that constantly having to make decisions will degrade our ability to make good ones. And we've all experienced the "oh, who gives a crap?" feeling when we're mentally exhausted and just want to comfort ourselves with our favorite vice.

In the course of this book, we'll be looking at several ways to build willpower, just as if it were a muscle you drag to the gym three times a week. Both mindfulness and the concept of the fight-thru strengthen our resolve and increase the amount of temptation we can withstand.

But right now, our goal is to do away with the need for willpower entirely. And we can do that by making a decision once, and then never making it again.

The Powerlessness Model of Addiction

Glenn Livingston, author of *Never Binge Again*, takes issue with the mainstream theory of addiction, which says things like "once an addict, always an addict," and instructs people to take their struggle with addiction "one day at a time." This thinking, he argues, makes every single day into a hard battle to resist the temptation of alcohol abuse.

This thinking is codified in the first three steps of 12-Step programs: we're powerless over our addiction, we come to believe in a power greater than ourselves, and we turn our life over to that power to save us.

Now, if 12-Step programs work for you, that's great. They do help some people manage their addictions without constant relapse. I don't want to convince you otherwise.

But for the majority of people struggling with addictions, this underlying message of personal powerlessness actually undermines the thinking and DOing required for full mastery over our habits and behaviors.

Lean on Character, Not Willpower

Instead of relying on willpower, Glenn recommends leaning on character. And the way to do this is to make a one-time decision and then stop deciding.

As in, "I don't eat cookies, cupcakes, cake, donuts, croissants, ice cream, or any form of recreational sugar. Ever."

Or, "I always drink 16 ounces of water when I wake up in the morning."

When you make a decision, a real decision, then other options are off the table. The word *decide* comes from the same Latin root as *incise* and *homicide*, meaning to cut off or to kill. Deciding means cutting off or killing the possibilities you've decided against.

Once you decide that you don't eat recreational sugar, then cookies and ice cream are no longer an option. You don't have to count the days since your last binge or wonder about the days until your next one. You don't have to agonize about whether to reject the dessert menu every time you go out to eat with friends.

Once you decide that you drink 16 ounces of water upon waking, you don't have to waffle about whether you're going to start your day with two glasses of water.

That kind of commitment sound scary? Well, it can be. But that's because you're pushing yourself to evolve into someone you're not used to. And change is scary. But you don't get something without giving something else up. So, you DO it because you decided to DO it. And that's that.

How Do You Keep Not Robbing That Bank?

When Glenn Livingston's clients talk about the constant pull of temptation and bring up the research on willpower being a limited resource (which lets them off the hook, because, hey, you can only do so many pushups before your muscles give out, right?), Glenn stops them in their tracks with a question:

"Do you rob banks?"

Confused, they answer, "No, of course not." (So far no one has admitted to being a bank robber.)

Glenn goes on: "Do you pass a bank on a regular basis?"

They generally answer yes, there's a bank where they shop, or on the way to work, or somewhere else nearby and convenient.

Then Glenn hits them with the kicker: "How do you resist the temptation to walk into the lobby, hand the teller a note, and steal all the money?"

They always respond that there's no temptation to do that, and so nothing to resist.

At this point Glenn explains that at some point in their life, they made a character decision not to rob banks. They probably didn't do it consciously, with a spreadsheet full of pros and cons, but they still made it. They decided that they were not the sort of person who robs banks.

And from that day forward, there was absolutely zero willpower required to walk past a bank and not rush in and shout, "Everybody on the floor. This is a holdup."

The trick to willpower when it comes to your health behaviors is *not needing any*, because you've made a similarly binding decision. You can then walk past a Little Debby Snack Cake or bottle of Jim Beam without any internal drama or ego depletion or decision fatigue.

Decisions are Vows

For most of us, decisions are wimpy things that we can go back on at any time. And for lots of decisions, that's not a big deal. There's no real cost to reversing them.

Due to a constant barrage of advertising, many of our decisions are couched in brand terms. Android or Apple. Ram or F-150 or Silverado. Crest or Colgate. And while you may have strong opinions about these choices, they don't really matter very much in the big picture of our lives.

But our health and lifestyle and ethical decisions are different. And when we approach them like consumers choosing toothpaste, it's no wonder we vacillate and backslide and constantly battle temptation.

So let's imbue our real decisions with gravity, and treat them differently from the daily choices that don't ultimately determine our destiny.

Let's call them vows.

Vows, unlike decisions, are sacred. In order to be a person of character, you instinctively want to honor your vows.

Glenn points out that he's never heard a marriage vow that goes, "I promise to be faithful to you unless somebody hotter comes along," or "I'm 80% sure that I won't cheat on you." (And while marriage vows obviously get broken, they still serve to stabilize the institution most of the time.)

So as you discover the habits and choices and rules that support your desired goals, turn the big ones into sacred vows. Make the decision once, and then never struggle with decision fatigue again.

You may still feel the craving, but that's different from having to make the decision again and again, every time the temptation presents itself. And as research shows, cravings that aren't fed quickly subside and soon go away.

So as you begin your Big Change journey, practice keeping your word to yourself. You can start small, with decisions that are easy for you to uphold.

You already do this much more than you think. You put on your seatbelt every time you get in a car, right? Even if you're in a rush, or you've got a cup of coffee in one hand.

Notice where in your life you're operating from unconscious vows, or character decisions that are no longer negotiable.

Then, on that foundation of success, add one new vow. Make it small and easy to keep. But keep it as if your life depended on it.

Because in a real way, it does. The ability to trust your own word is the basis of a successful Big Change.

5

GET THE NAQ: ONE IDEA TO RULE THEM ALL

Now that you know where you're going (the big promise of Chapter 1) and met your guides (Chapter 2)—plus inoculated yourself against early-stage self-sabotage (Chapter 3) and fired up the three engines of change (Chapter 4)—it's time to look at the map and plan your route.

In this chapter, you'll discover the Big Idea that will guide your thinking as you build the three pillars of Big Change: Menu, Movement, and Mindset.

Ready? Cool.

Naturally Attainable Quantities (NAQ)

In a landscape full of competing theories, claims, and hype, how do we know what we should be eating to be lean, energetic, and healthy?

In a confusing shout-fest of contradictory fitness advice, how can we tell what exercises we should be doing, and for how long, at what intervals, and at what level of intensity?

In a self-help world populated by self-appointed experts and myopic researchers clinging to their one original idea, how do we know what modes of thinking best serve us, our goals, and our happiness?

In other words, is there a litmus test that we can apply across the board to figure out whether a piece of advice makes sense or is probably nonsense?

Yes. That litmus test is a simple question: "What is the naturally attainable quantity of a particular food in a traditional and sustainable human society?"

The answer to that question tells us how much of something human beings evolved to get. How much we're designed to get. How much we can handle. And how much we need.

It's a very simple concept, and one we can wield with incredible power to cut through the confusion. Food is the foundation of human civilization; once we know what we're meant to eat, and how much, then we can extrapolate the Movement and exertion that would have been required to attain it. And the Mindsets and habits that would have supported that level of effort.

To get the NAQ, picture yourself in our ancestors' natural environment: no fancy technologies or minions at your beck and call. No motors, no engines, no batteries, no hierarchies of labor, no classes of workers, and no stealing of tomorrow's resources to get through today.

What types and volumes of food could you acquire? What amount of physical Movement and exertion would be required? How much discomfort would you have to endure?

NAQ and Sudoku: Finding a Single Right Answer

What NAQ really does is answer the question, "Does this idea make sense?" Because there's an awful lot of nonsense out there.

Consider the piece of advice we hear over and over again, "Eat less, move more." Or, to be slightly more science-y about it, "Reduce your energy intake (calories) so it's lower than your energy expenditure (exercise)."

That formulation gives us a lot of leeway. As long as we find a way to balance inputs and outputs, the theory goes, we're doing fine. But when you start looking at it in practice, it doesn't quite hang together.

An Olympic swimmer like Michael Phelps is balancing input and output when he eats 10,000 calories of donuts, pizza, and fried chicken and works out in a 60 degree pool for five hours a day. And he's not overweight, is he? So everything must be cool. Except when we look at the shape of his arteries, and what science tells us about his long-term health prospects, that diet is far from optimal.

Think of all the different diet and exercise options as a completely blank Sudoku grid. It's got a trillion trillion possible solutions (the exact number is 6,670,903,752,021,072,936,960, according to Wikipedia). You could spend the rest of your life constructing unique 9x9 grids according to the rules of Sudoku and never complete them all; it would take millennia. That's what it can feel like when you're trying to puzzle out how to eat and move and think in a healthy way: overwhelming and pointless.

But the puzzles you see in the newspapers and in-flight magazines, with a few numbers pre-filled, have only one correct answer. That's what happens when we apply NAQ to the Menu question.

Not only do we get a clear and common-sense answer for Menu, it also allows us to answer the Movement and Mindset questions correctly.

How to Apply NAQ

Let's apply NAQ to Menu, and then see how it fills in all the other Sudoku squares.

Menu

Menu, or the food we eat, is the foundation of Big Change.

You simply can't be healthy and happy if your diet isn't right. I don't care how powerful your Ferrari Berlinetta is; if you pour Diet

Pepsi or dirty cooking oil into the fuel tank, that vehicle isn't going anywhere.

You can't out-exercise a bad diet. And no matter how positive your thinking, when you eat substances not fit for human consumption (which is pretty much what most Americans eat, most of the time), your mind and mood will eventually succumb to biological reality: they can't operate well in the absence of fiber and the presence of chronically inflammatory chemicals that characterize the standard American diet.

So what should humans eat? We'll get into that in detail in the Menu chapter. For right now, let's practice applying the NAQ to the foods we eat by looking at three examples: cow's milk, Nabisco Nutter Butter cookies, and lean chicken breast.

Cow's Milk

Even as an adult human who had been weaned decades earlier, I (Josh) would think nothing of polishing off multiple gallons of milk a day. When I was running around in my truck, taking care of the trailer park and maintaining my pump stations, I would reward myself at the gas station convenience store with a half-gallon of milk and a package of Nutter Butters.

The Nutter Butters were an indulgence, granted, but I was sure I was nourishing my giant human body with the white liquid.

After all: Got milk? It does a body good. It builds bones. It makes athletes big and strong, especially when poured over a bowl of Wheaties. The government even makes sure that every child in America has access to milk every day at school. I was just being a responsible adult by drinking that excellent source of calcium and protein.

Let's give milk the NAQ treatment and see how it shakes out.

In a traditional human society, our infants were nourished exclusively by human breast milk for the first year or so of life. Hunter-gatherer babies nursed for approximately 4-5 years, and then never drank dairy again. There simply was no way for a human to reliably source the breast milk of another mammal.

As we moved into animal husbandry, there might have been a cow or goat who had a little excess milk after providing for her calf or kid. That milk, available a couple months at a time in small amounts, would have supplemented the diets of humans and provided a concentrated source of fat and protein. But because grazing animals compete with cropland, which feed humans much more efficiently than animal agriculture, the amount of spare milk available would have been a negligible part of any one person's diet.

The idea that a cup of cow's milk three times a day is a naturally attainable quantity is ridiculous. And don't get us started on cheese, which concentrates the milk up to 100 times. The amount of cheese slathered on the average pizza slice represents gallons and gallons of milk – the opposite of NAQ. This concentrates the casomorphins (addictive mood-altering compounds) that nature put in milk so that infants get hooked on nursing from the first moments of life.

And you wonder why a lot of people say they'd rather die than give up cheese? They're chemically addicted, that's why.

Nutter Butter Cookies

Obviously, there were no such things as Nutter Butters in a traditional human society, but we can still do the mental exercise we did for cow's milk by examining Nutter Butters' component ingredients. These include, in descending weight order, white wheat flour, sugar, peanuts, corn syrup, and several kinds of vegetable oil (mostly hydrogenated or partly hydrogenated rapeseed, cottonseed, soybean, peanut, canola, and palm).

Humans domesticated wheat a couple thousand years ago, but the area of wheat required to produce a box of Nutter Butters would have been several square feet, since our ancestors wouldn't have been able to add synthetic fertilizer, pesticides, herbicides, and fungicides. And the genetic manipulation that allows for wheat's current intense growing and easy harvest is recent, with the most significant advances occurring since the 1970s.

The sugar in a full package of Nutter Butters would have required a couple of sugar canes, or several pounds of beets, depending on the source, although a traditional society wouldn't have had the means to refine the sugar to anywhere close to the purity of today's white crystals.

The peanuts needed might have grown in a 3-foot section of garden bed, say 4 robust plants. The high fructose corn syrup would have required several corn plants, and maybe up to half a bushel of corn (though, again, the manufacturing process would have been far out of our ancestors' capability, without synthetic chemicals and factories driven by fossil fuel power). And the oils, even if non-hydrogenated, would be so wasteful that no traditional society would have dreamed of sacrificing precious nuts, beans, seeds, or palm fruit just to extract them.

The Nutter Butter verdict? There's no way they would have existed at all in a traditional human diet. If you're going eat them in naturally attainable quantities, you're not going to eat them. If you still must, they should be a rare treat at best.

Lean Chicken Breast

Hey, this is a health food, right? Low fat, full of protein, and part of every good athlete's diet. When I (Josh) tried to lose weight before I understood NAQ, I would gorge myself on chicken breasts and then go lift weights. Man-food!

So let's subject lean chicken breast to some NAQ scrutiny: What's the naturally attainable quantity of chicken for a human being living in our environment, without the use of fossil fuels or other people's labor?

Without those things, we don't have giant factory farms raising tens of billions of chickens per year. We don't have synthetic fertilizers that grow immense fields of grain and soybeans to feed to those chickens. We don't have the capacity to pump millions of gallons of groundwater from aquifers to clean out the chicken housing and dilute their waste. We don't have industrial quantities of antibiotics that make the chickens gain weight far beyond what is natural for their species.

We don't have trains and trucks to ship feed to the chicken factories or transport the dead chickens to our grocery stores. And we don't have grocery stores, or refrigeration, so we can't easily store it in mass quantities for whenever we want.

In other words, we don't have a steady, virtually unlimited supply of chicken to eat on a daily basis.

Instead, we occasionally hunt for wild fowl (which has very little fat). We can eat only what we can catch locally. And our ecosystem can support only so many of these wild birds per acre; if we catch and kill them all, our meat-eating isn't sustainable.

Or we might practice animal husbandry, keeping as many chickens as we can feed from our own kitchen scraps and fields and gardens and woodlots. That number will be tiny indeed, as we can't farm enough land to feed all those animals and ourselves. It's about 10 times more efficient to eat corn than to feed that corn to a chicken and eat the chicken. Eating chicken more than a few times a year simply isn't sustainable for humans living in a traditional society.

The only way we are able to consume chicken on a daily basis is through the twin engines of fossil fuels and tens of thousands of low-paid workers—who end up suffering from debilitating health conditions caused by their exposure to sick, drugged-up chickens. (Not-so-fun fact: men who work in chicken processing plants get cancer of the penis at a rate nine times higher than the general male population. You can look it up: http://bit.ly/penis-cancer. Also the rates of just about every other kind of cancer are higher among chicken processing plant workers as well: http://bit.ly/all-cancers.)

Clearly, these inputs aren't sustainable. Over time, they degrade our environment, damage the health of workers and communities living near the chicken factories, and use up land that could otherwise be deployed in ways that improve human life.

So when someone tells you that humans are designed to drink

lots of milk, eat Nutter Butters "in moderation," or consume chicken breast on a daily basis, you can run those claims through the NAQ filter and see them for the nonsense they are.

Movement

Even if we might quibble over some of the calculations, it makes sense to talk about food in terms of NAQ. But how can we translate Movement into quantities?

Basically, animals move in order to survive.

If you're a predator, you move to catch your prey. If you're the prey, you move to escape.

If you're an herbivore, you move to cover your territory to graze.

And animals move to avoid bad weather, to compete in the quest for mates, to provide for their young, and to mark their territories.

For the human animal in traditional society, these Movement requirements were just that: requirements. Not optional.

We didn't have internal combustion engines that used the carcasses of dinosaurs to power vehicles into the savanna when we went hunting.

We didn't have Amazon Dash buttons to reorder Pringles, Gatorade, and Doritos without leaving the house.

And we didn't have the military or economic power to compel millions of people around the world to grow our sugar and coffee and beef in place of their own subsistence crops.

So let's fill in the Movement Sudoku square with the type, amount, intensity, frequency, and nature of physical exertion that would have been required of a human being living in our environment.

Call it our Movement MED: Minimum Exertion Demanded.

The primary type of human Movement, of course, is bipedal locomotion. As in walking, jogging, running.

It drives us nuts when people say, "Oh, I'm not a runner." Imagine an oriole saying, "Oh, I'm not really a flyer." Or a halibut going, "Yeah,

I'm not crazy about swimming. Hurts my fins." Or a kangaroo insisting — you get the idea.

Humans walk and run. To collect resources. To avoid dangers and discomforts. Sometimes they walk in a leisurely fashion, and sometimes they haul ass. Whatever the MED.

Sometimes they get to rest and recover between bouts of intense Movement, and sometimes they have no choice but to power through despite extreme soreness and fatigue. Sometimes the MED is quite a lot, if they want to survive a rough patch.

Our existence is proof our ancestors did those things. So if we think of our 45 minutes a day of cardio as "optional," we're completely disregarding hundreds of thousands of years of hominid evolution.

We didn't just walk or run, of course. We also lifted objects, heavy and light. We climbed. We jumped. We pushed and pulled. We twisted.

We weren't Movement specialists, spending hours on treadmills or sitting on benches moving steel plates up and down. We had to engage with our messy, variable, unpredictable environments and grow our muscles, tendons, and lung capacity to handle whatever challenge life threw at us next.

Kind of the ultimate CrossFit, without the t-shirt.

Mindset

Now that we've established how we would have gathered and prepared our food, built or found shelter, and defended ourselves, our families, and our territories from predators, we can also fill in the Sudoku squares of Mindset.

We can split our discussion of Mindset into two particularly relevant topics: Discomfort and Presence.

Embrace Discomfort

There are things we are able to avoid in our modern, industrialized culture that simply wouldn't have been an option to avoid in a traditional society. Pretty much anything that makes us physically uncomfortable can be escaped: cold, hunger, wet, heat, humidity, biting insects, muscle soreness, etc.

And we have turned comfort into something that must be sought at all costs. As Marc Schoen, PhD, points out in *Your Survival Instinct Is Killing You*, most of us are so obsessed with avoiding discomfort that we drive ourselves crazy worrying about it. And the more comfortable we get, paradoxically, the more stressed out we become at the thought of discomfort.

If you never feel cold, thanks to indoor heating, then the thought of being caught outdoors in the snow can be terrifying. If you do everything in your power to not have uncomfortable conversations with family members, friends, and colleagues, then the mere possibility of having to raise an awkward issue can clamp your mouth shut. The longer you reside in your comfort zone, the scarier it feels to venture outside of it.

So let's consider: how much discomfort would be required of us in a traditional society? In order to move as much as we needed to do all the things we talked about in the last section, including finding food?

Answer: Plenty.

We have evolved as a species not only to be able to withstand environmental stressors, but to actually require them to be healthy. In that regard, we are what philosopher Nassim Nicholas Taleb calls "antifragile" in his book of that name, getting stronger rather than weaker from stress and uncertainty.

Unless we intentionally expose ourselves to cold, heat, and hunger on an intermittent basis, we weaken in body and mind.

Unless we push ourselves into the kind of physical exertion that makes our heart pound, our skin sweat, and our muscles ache, we grow listless and emotionally unbalanced.

We call this "Vitamin PD," for productive discomfort. We ask each other, "Did you get your Vitamin PD today?"

Vitamin PD comes in mental and emotional form, as well as physical. It means having difficult conversations, embracing conflict, sitting with anger, sadness, guilt, and shame, instead of distracting ourselves with technology or numbing out with food, drugs, and porn.

We want to challenge ourselves and push our boundaries, not cause lasting harm to our bodies and minds. So along with Vitamin PD comes a clear exhortation to know yourself—your limits, your tendency to push too hard or not hard enough, and your own body's pain signals.

The goal of Vitamin PD is a better life, not a worse one.

Cultivate Presence

We also want to cultivate the quality of Presence. Being here now. Focusing on the situation at hand, without reliving the past or worrying about the future. We can't embrace discomfort if we're not able to cultivate an ability to focus our attention on the here and now.

It's no secret that our technologies, though wonderful in so many ways, have created a society in which we're constantly distracted. We can tune out of the here and now at any time, by virtue of our smartphones. Just Google "Venice gondola smartphone" to view the viral video of a gondola riding down a canal in Venice with four tourists staring at their phones, completely missing the wonders all around them.

But even without access to pocket technology, we humans are really good at being Anywhere But Here.

That simply did not work in our ancestral NAQ environment. For one thing, we would never survive predators if we didn't constantly scan our surroundings for signs of danger. For another, we would starve if we weren't attuned to the subtle clues that signal the presence of potential food sources.

Paying attention is one form of presence. Another is what we might call meditation, or the ability to diffuse our attention and restore our nervous system to a peaceful, harmonious, resting state.

In our natural environment, we received cues to reset our nervous system on a daily basis: sunsets, vistas, oceans, birdsong, organic smells such as turpenes from trees and geosmin from soil bacteria (the latter responsible for that wonderful scent of the earth after a rain).

But in a high-tech world (by which we also mean technologies like indoor spaces, artificial lighting, and pavement), we're deprived of all those cues that heal our jangled nerves.

So in order to achieve regular doses of Meditation — of Presence — we have to practice it, schedule it and commit to it.

The Golden Rule: Pace Yourself

Now that we've explored the NAQ of Menu and the MED of Movement, and how both relate to Mindset, we're ready to dive into the details in the following chapters.

But there are two more things you need to know before we dive into the details of Big Change.

The first is: Go at your own pace.

There's no timeline written in stone for how long it will take you to lose 20 pounds, or be free of a particular craving, or run a mile in 12 minutes.

When we compare ourselves to others and to "objective" standards of progress, we invariably make ourselves miserable inside and out.

Your body is unique, as is your history of taking care of it (and failing to take care of it).

You may have particular health challenges. You may have tons of family or work responsibilities. You may have more or less money with which to buy time or gear.

You may be naturally optimistic or pessimistic.

You may live near the ocean with access to fresh tropical fruit and the gentle sound of surf, or in a polluted inner city with toxic drinking water and the constant wails of sirens.

There's no basis for comparison with anyone else.

So set your goals, and be both fierce and gentle with yourself.

Focus on DOing rather than outcome. If your DOing doesn't bring you closer to your desired outcome, remember the Results Dictate Sufficiency engine. DO more. DO less. DO different. Tweak, experiment, observe, and repeat.

The Other Golden Rule: Find Community

Even though comparisons are toxic, finding a community of Changers is crucial. It's almost impossible to be successful on this journey all by yourself.

Our culture is designed to get you to eat crappy food, be sedentary, and drown your sorrows with consumption. If you don't intentionally seek out the company (in person and virtually) of people who are also choosing a different life, you'll spend all your time swimming upstream. Eventually you'll exhaust yourself, and most likely give up.

Look for local hiking meet-ups and running groups.

Seek out communities where people gather around healthy cooking and eating, or start your own monthly potlucks.

And join our Sick to Fit Facebook community, where you'll find many like-minded people on a similar journey, happy to share encouragement, guidance, a well-timed kick in the ass, and laughter and commiseration.

Remember, you can find it at Facebook.com/groups/sicktofit. We look forward to meeting you there.

6

MENU

O K, now it's time to dive into the nuts and bolts of Big Change. As you've seen, we've identified three fundamental aspects, the "pillars" of Big Change: Menu, Movement, and Mindset.

Each of them builds on and reinforces the others, but you don't have to address them in any particular order; Josh started with Movement, while Howard began with Menu. However, if we did have to choose the most crucial one, it would be Menu: the food we put in our mouths every day.

Here's why, by way of a cliché we don't stop to think about enough: "You are what you eat."

The food we consume literally turns into us, into the tissues and cells of our bodies. It also gets converted into the energy that powers your every step and your every thought. So however you're moving and whatever you're thinking, it's energy from your food that's doing the moving and thinking.

In this section, we're going to cover three main topics:

1. What to eat — the details of the dietary style best suited to human health, fitness, and happiness.

2. How to transition to this diet — the approaches and potential pitfalls on your transformation journey.
3. Transition tools — the specific strategies and skills that you'll need in order to be fully successful.

With Josh as your guide, let's get started...

What to Eat

Everything I'm going to say here is ultimately based on the key concept of Naturally Attainable Quantities (NAQ), but it's also backed up by the preponderance of scientific evidence.

This isn't a science book, so I'm not going to try to convince you that this way of eating is based on evidence by sharing studies and facts and biochemical pathways.

If you want or need that kind of reassurance before committing, then here are some resources that I depend on for the facts about nutrition and health:

- NutritionFacts.org, the website of Michael Greger, MD, which has thousands of short videos that examine research studies on nutrition. Also check out his year-in-review presentations on big topics, like the 15 leading causes of death and disability, and his series on specific foods like eggs and poultry.
- *The China Study*, and *Whole*, by T. Colin Campbell, PhD. The most highly respected nutrition researcher in the world, Campbell's findings have revolutionized our understanding of how to prevent cancer, heart disease, and other chronic conditions through our food choices. Also, Howard co-wrote *Whole*, which is how I first heard of him.
- *Proteinaholic*, by Garth Davis, MD. Garth (he's become a good buddy, so I get to be on a first-name basis with him) is both a practicing general and bariatric surgeon, and

incredible researcher. This book (also with an assist by Howard) references 700 published studies, and teaches readers how to understand and interpret the evidence, plus how to defend against the nutritional nonsense that's all around us.

With that out of the way, let's talk about what to eat. I'll explain the qualities of the foods we want to eat, then the quantities, and finally look at the specific foods that make up my diet.

Qualities

The ideal Menu is made up of unprocessed plant foods that are calorically dilute and multi-colored. Let's break that down.

Unprocessed plant foods

According to the theory of NAQ, humans have evolved to get about 95% of our calories from plants. I know that the Paleo folks are all into the mythology of "man as hunter," but when you think about it, you quickly realize that any human in danger of starvation would prefer a harmless, stationary, colorful sure thing of a plant to a potentially violent, fast-moving, camouflaged gamble of an animal. While meat was certainly an opportunistic part of the human diet, we are designed to be plant-eaters first and foremost.

Not only that, but we evolved to eat *unprocessed* plant foods: vegetables, fruits, whole grains, tubers, legumes, and nuts and seeds in as close to their natural state as possible. Not processed food fragments (like corn syrup, wheat flour, olive oil). And not adulterated with additives and preservatives and flavorings, but comprised solely of natural ingredients.

Clarification

Bear in mind that, even when we aim for 100% perfection,

we realize we won't achieve it 100% of the time. We live in an imperfect world, and we have to make allowances from time to time. The big goal here is to make our Menu predominantly unprocessed plant food. If our daily normal is healthy, then, for most of us, some occasional and limited deviations will not be a big deal for most of us.

If you've got heart disease, cancer, type II diabetes, or an autoimmune disease or other condition that's extremely sensitive to diet, like an allergy, then of course 100% compliance may be your only responsible option. But that's your call.

Calorically dilute

The second quality we're seeking in our Menu is foods low in caloric density. That is, we want to fill our stomachs as full as possible with the fewest number of calories.

Back when I was a fat guy, I specialized in volume eating. I loved to fill my belly with as large a quantity of food as possible. If you also have that tendency, then choosing calorically dilute foods as the bulk of your diet will be crucial for weight loss.

Our body's first signal of fullness comes from the stomach's stretch receptors. And again, this is the NAQ at work. The human default in our natural environment was to guard against starvation. So we would always eat as much as we could get our hands on to make sure we consumed enough calories to power our efforts to find more food down the line. And since the foods that were most common and most accessible tended to be the most calorically dilute, like leafy greens, tubers, fruits, and vegetables, we had to eat for volume just to take in enough energy to survive.

Caloric Density

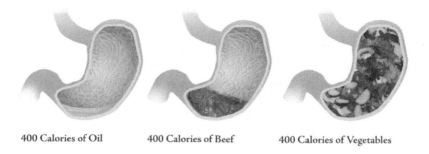

400 Calories of Oil   400 Calories of Beef   400 Calories of Vegetables

Stretch receptors are located throughout the stomach. When they are triggered by food, they send signals to your brain to tell you to stop eating. With high fiber, whole plant foods, you can eat the most quantity for the least amount of calories.

© 2012 Julieanna Hever, MS, RD, CPT • www.PlantBasedDietitian.com
Illustration by Sherri Nestorowich • www.sherrinest.wix.com/art

Here's a picture of how the same number of calories of different foods affect our stomach's stretch receptors that says a thousand words, courtesy of dietitian Julieanna Hever:

Now that we live in a world of 24/7 access to calorie-dense foods that never existed in nature (think of those Nutter Butters from the last chapter, at 2100 calories per pound, or bacon, at 2000 calories per pound), we have to be extra vigilant to mimic our NAQ of these foods.

Chef AJ of EatUnprocessed.com created the figure below to make caloric density simple. It's a continuum, with the least dense foods on the left and the most dense on the right.

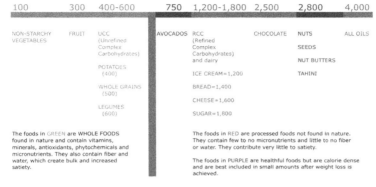

CHEF AJ's **CALORIE DENSITY CHART**
Average calories per pound

100	300	400-600	750	1,200-1,800	2,500	2,800	4,000
NON-STARCHY VEGETABLES	FRUIT	UCC (Unrefined Complex Carbohydrates)	AVOCADOS	RCC (Refined Complex Carbohydrates) and dairy	CHOCOLATE	NUTS	ALL OILS
						SEEDS	
						NUT BUTTERS	
		POTATOES (400)		ICE CREAM = 1,200		TAHINI	
		WHOLE GRAINS (500)		BREAD = 1,400			
		LEGUMES (600)		CHEESE = 1,600			
				SUGAR = 1,800			

The foods in GREEN are WHOLE FOODS found in nature and contain vitamins, minerals, antioxidants, phytochemicals and micronutrients. They also contain fiber and water, which create bulk and increased satiety.

The foods in RED are processed foods not found in nature. They contain few to no micronutrients and little to no fiber or water. They contribute very little to satiety.

The foods in PURPLE are healthful foods but are calorie dense and are best included in small amounts after weight loss is achieved.

For weight loss, weight management and optimum health:
EAT TO THE LEFT OF THE RED LINE.

www.eatunprocessed.com   Copyright 2017 - Chef AJ's Healthy Kitchen LLC

AJ draws a red vertical line at the about 550 calories per pound mark. Her one rule for weight loss: Eat to the left of the red line. That is, eat foods that have lots of volume (to trigger our stomach stretch receptors' message of "Stop eating; you're full!") and not so many calories.

As you can see, that translates to a diet of non-starchy vegetables, fruit, and unrefined complex carbohydrates. Once you've achieved your ideal weight, you can start adding in small amounts of calorically dense but still healthy plant-based foods like nuts, seeds, and avocados.

Rainbow of colors

Third, our Menu should contain a rainbow of different colors. I'm not talking about Skittles, obviously, but the real red of tomatoes, orange of carrots, yellow-orange of cantaloupe, green of kale, blue of blueberries, indigo of eggplant, violet of purple potatoes, white of onions, and so on.

It's not just that eating a rainbow keeps us from getting bored. Different colors of plant foods provide specific nutrients, so eating a diversity of colors ensures we get a diversity of nutrients.

I suspect that's why we have color vision: to enable us to go to the pharmacy of nature and grab the right medicine for what's going on. As an example, Michael Greger, MD, of NutritionFacts.org points to the benefits of different color foods for different aspects of vision: green pigment in food is protective against glaucoma, while yellow helps prevent macular degeneration.

So whenever you have the choice, select a rainbow, and look for intense, saturated colors rather than washed out pastels. Go for those tomatoes, deep red onions, purple or orange sweet potatoes (they're amazing just done in the microwave), broccoli slaw, all colors of bell peppers, and the like.

A lot of diets involve tortuous calculations and obsessive micromanagement of macronutrients (carbohydrates, fats, and protein). But the great news is, we don't have to worry about that when we follow the three Menu guidelines and eat plant foods that are minimally processed, calorically dilute, and in a rainbow of colors. Let everyone else obsess about macronutrient ratios. Turns out that, when we focus on the quality of our food (via the lens of NAQ), macronutrients take care of themselves.

Quantities

I know this is the Menu section, but I have to bring Movement in for just a minute. Because everything here is connected, and nowhere is that clearer than when we think about the link between the quantity of food we eat and the energy we expend in the world.

There has to be an energy balance between Menu and Movement.

It's simple, really: if you're moving around a lot, you'll need a lot more calories. If you're not moving much, your calorie quantity should go down.

A few months ago I was coming off an injury, and was unable to run. I would swim, go on the elliptical in the gym, and DO some pushups and other calisthenics, but it definitely wasn't the equivalent of my 60+ mile weeks with an average pace of 8 or 9 minutes per mile. So I consciously ate a lot less than I normally would have.

There's a common misconception that you can just eat whatever you want on a NAQ diet and you don't need to exercise at all. That's often true at the beginning of your weight loss journey, especially if you're starting out really heavy, like I was. I know plenty of fat people who started gorging on whole plant foods and dropped 50-100 pounds pretty much by accident while not restricting quantities at all.

It's easy to see why when you think about caloric density: all of a sudden that stomach that used to get filled up with 4000 calories is now getting equally full from 600 calories.

But there's going to come a time when that effortless weight loss is going to stop, and you're going to have to adjust your quantities of food intake based on your Movement requirements.

Again, the reason comes down to the whole NAQ thing. Every animal in nature obtains its food by scurrying around, swimming, flying, slithering, or some other form of Movement. And in nature, the more you move, the more calories you both need and get. Some animals, like predators, expend huge amounts of energy, and so they require lots of calories — which make it convenient that they're meat eaters, naturally sourcing those calories from their prey, who concentrate them from the plants *they* eat.

It's a very efficient system, and it's worked for millions of years. Every animal alive today comes equipped with evolutionary mechanisms that match the environment in which its ancestors evolved, where its default Movement and default Menu are in dynamic equilibrium.

The problem with humans today is that our evolutionary environment is gone. Our modern society has upset that balance. Instead of eating plants and moving like predators, we move like plants and eat like predators. So in order to be healthy organisms of appropriate weight, we have to simulate that environment through our choices and behaviors.

Even if you're eating a 100% whole food, plant-based diet, you can't eat dates stuffed with peanut butter all day and lose weight. (I tell you this from experience!)

Back to NAQ

When you're thinking about how much of a particular food to eat, fall back on NAQ.

If a food is on the far left of Chef AJ's chart, the extremely calorically dilute category, eat all you want. For humans, leafy greens, broccoli, cauliflower, and cabbage are pretty much a free-for-all. Keep some of that raw to simulate the amount of chewing our ancestors would have had to do, and you're golden.

Next comes fruit, which, when it's in season, is abundant, accessible, and visually arresting. Go wild – eat as much as you like.

Slightly, but not much higher in calories per pound are foods like tubers and legumes and whole grains. You can eat as much as you want from these categories (if you wanted to live exclusively on potatoes, for example, you'd have to eat around six pounds a day to get enough calories to function), as long as you don't process the life (and water and fiber) out of them or drown them in salt, sugar, and oil.

The most calorically dense foods typically require the most time and effort to procure and prepare. It's easy to consume 7500 calories in pecans from a giant Costco bag, but if you have a pecan tree, you know that grabbing even a handful of pecans requires great patience and effort.

First, you have to beat the squirrels to the nuts. Second, you have to store them for six to nine months until they start tasting good (the nuts, not the squirrels). Third, you have to crack them open. Try it without technology more advanced than two rocks and you'll quickly see what kind of time and effort we're talking about. Fourth, about a quarter of the pecans will be rotten. And finally, you have to separate the nut meat from the shell bits before eating.

All told, it requires about six months of waiting and half an hour's hard labor for 100 calories of pecans. That's a naturally attainable quantity. So while nuts are technically whole, plant-based foods, you'll want to limit yourself to a small handful a day, unless your physical activity level mimics the effort it would take to gather larger quantities (if you're an endurance athlete, say, or a Paleolithic re-enactor).

Seasonality

In addition to asking how much of this food you could source from nature, also think about how often and when you could get it.

If you live in a temperate climate, fruits are abundant for part of the year. I'll eat lots of watermelon during the summer, but I won't have much in December. Two whole watermelons a day might be naturally attainable for a span of a few weeks, and indulging then makes sense because leaner times are on their way. In our modern world, we can purchase the bounty of summer fruits all through the year, which is decidedly unnatural.

Our level of Movement also changed with the seasons back in the day, as different weather and availability of food dictated different survival strategies. Of course, we didn't have to figure all this out – Menu and Movement just came naturally. Now, we have to use our heads to imitate what used to be instinctive responses to our environments.

Specific Foods

Now that we've got the theory covered, let's see where the rhubarb meets the road. I'll tell you about how I shop and what I eat in a typical week.

I'm not saying it's the best way to do things, and it's definitely not the only one, but it works for me. And it doesn't require special cooking skills, or tons of time, or—now that I've become good at it—even the ability to think ahead very much. But I want to share it as an example of "If I can DO it, then you definitely can."

I divide my food shopping into three categories: weekly grocery store trips where I fill up a cart, daily "top-up" trips for ingredients for fresh meals, and "extreme food shopping" when I'm on the road and all I can find is a gas station, convenience store, or even a rural bait and tackle shop hundreds of miles from the nearest Whole Foods.

Makin' Groceries

"Makin' Groceries" is bayou-speak for a trip to the grocery store where you push around a cart and bring home a big pile of stuff. You probably call it "going grocery shopping."

Now, the way I "make groceries" is almost certainly going to be different from the way you do it. For one thing, my wife and I don't have kids, and you might.

For another, I try to keep things really simple, both in terms of taste and preparation. You see, I used to be addicted not only to vast quantities of unhealthy food, but also to my identity as "the chef." I was always the one getting hugs and kisses for my speckled trout, barbecued ribs, and massive pots of gumbo, and that identity as an obsessive foodie fueled my dysfunctional relationship with food.

Lots of vegans love preparing fancy dishes to show that plants can be just as delicious as meat and dairy. I get where they're coming from, but I have no use for complicated recipes (or recipes of any kind, for that matter). Food is fuel, not entertainment. The fact that whole plant foods taste delicious is just a bonus.

For a third, I'm on the road most of the day, so I don't really have a set time when I can spend even half an hour in the kitchen. I rely on my electric pressure cooker: fill it in the morning, eat from it in the evening. (Most recent models automatically switch from pressure cooking to "keep warm" mode, so you don't have to be home to babysit your dinner.) And lunch is usually in my truck on the way from one emergency to another, so it's gotta be finger food like apples, grapes, raw broccoli, carrots, cauliflower, and other produce I can eat without needing a table and cutlery and place setting.

I'm telling you all this so you don't go and unthinkingly copy my way of making groceries if it doesn't fit your lifestyle, preferences, priorities, or goals. I'm just being as transparent as possible about how I do food shopping, so you can visualize a clear example of what NAQ eating looks like; take what's useful and relevant for you, but focus on the principles rather than the details.

Since I don't do a ton of cooking, I focus my big shopping trips on gathering lots of prepared, bagged, and frozen foods. But if you have access to a farmers' market or love to cook, you can always substitute fresh, local, organic produce for the frozen and prepared stuff I get.

The Produce Section

Produce — fresh fruits and vegetables — is the basis of all my meals. Here are the categories of produce that I buy on my grocery runs:

Greens

The main ones I get are collards, mustard greens, Swiss chard, kale, and spinach. Most of my meals start with a big bowl of greens that other stuff gets piled onto. If you're shopping for a few days at a time, kale tends to last longer in the fridge than the others. I especially like lacinato or "dinosaur" kale for its ability to stay fresh and not wilt or get slimy.

Tubers

Basically, these are potatoes (russets, red potatoes, and Yukon gold) and sweet potatoes. They are very satisfying, not nearly as calorically dense as processed starches like bread or pasta, and keep well. I eat these pretty much every day.

The easiest way to consume tubers is to steam or boil them in the electric pressure cooker, or heat them in a microwave oven, and then mash them over a big bowl of greens. Sweet potatoes and dinosaur kale, red potatoes and mustard greens — you can vary the combination based on taste and availability. The heat from the potatoes wilts the greens just enough that they lose their raw edge, but don't get fully cooked. Science tells us that some valuable nutrients are lost in the cooking process, so eating close-to-raw greens confers some health benefits.

Cruciferous Vegetables

I'm going for convenience here, so I'll pick up a few bags of pre-cut broccoli or cauliflower florets, or bags of shredded cabbage, broccoli slaw, or cauliflower rice. I just toss this stuff into the pressure cooker with a legume — lentils or beans, see below — as part of a hearty vegetable stew, or in the case of the pre-cut vegetables, just eat them as finger food throughout the day.

Other Vegetables

Depending on what's available, I might grab some carrots, parsnips, summer or winter squash, tomatoes or eggplant for a pressure cooker stew.

Fresh Condiments

I often season my spuds and greens with salsa or pico de gallo, both made from tomatoes, onions, and herbs. I much prefer the kind sold in the produce section to the preserved jars in the center of the store. It's fresh-made, and much less adulterated, with few or no additives.

Fruit

I love Honeycrisp apples (most days, my lunch consists of three or four giant ones), grapes, bananas, mangoes, pears, and whatever else is in season, fresh, and delicious.

Dried foods

I shop sparingly from the rest of the supermarket, but there are a few staples that go along with my produce-heavy diet:

Grains

I'm talking whole, unprocessed grains here. I like barley, wheat berries, and brown rice. Rolled oats are good, but are slightly processed, and white rice, while not a whole food and therefore inferior to brown rice, is still acceptable if it's all you've got at the moment. I pick one grain, cook up a big pot, and add it to my stews for the next few meals. When it runs out, I'll repeat with a different grain.

Dried legumes

The legume family includes beans, peas, and lentils. I like lentils because they cook the fastest. Red lentils in particular will cook in a hurry, and turn into a soupy base for vegetables that is also delicious all by itself.

Condiments

I'm a big fan of nutritional yeast, which I sprinkle on most of my savory meals. I hate to run out, so I make sure to keep my pantry well stocked.

I use Tamari soy sauce sparingly, the low-sodium version if possible. Tamari is wheat- and often gluten-free, so it's a purer form of the condiment. But don't drown your food. If you skip the salt for a while to allow your sodium-addled taste buds to return to normal, after a few weeks or months the foods you used to add salt to will start tasting delicious without it. It's crazy how quickly our preferences reset to "normal" when we remove all the abnormally rich food from our Menus.

Another staple condiment in my house is Sriracha (Vietnamese "rooster" sauce). Some brands can be high in sugar, so I get the paste, which is less sweet and more concentrated.

Finally, I like mustard, which typically is one of the least adulterated of the store-bought condiments. Look for stone-ground mustard with few ingredients. Many mustards include turmeric, which is apparently some kind of health miracle substance. I just like the way it tastes.

Frozen Foods

Frozen produce is often as or more nutritious than fresh, especially if you're getting stuff that is grown across the country or across the world and spends days or weeks getting to you. Flash freezing retains lots of nutrients, requires less chemical manipulation to keep "fresh" in transit, and stores really well in your home as long as you have a decent freezer and working electricity. While using frozen food can conflict with the principle of eating in season, I'd rather you eat last summer's broccoli and cherries than last summer's wheat, cane sugar, and soybean oil.

Frozen Fruit

I love frozen fruit. I eat it like dessert, so I prefer fruit that is still "chewable" when frozen, like cherries, blueberries, mangos, and tropical fruit blends.

My wife has smoothies in the morning, so we go through bags of frozen bananas for those.

Frozen Aromatic Vegetables

In Louisiana we have what we call the "trinity" — onions, celery, and bell peppers — that we use as the base of our gumbos and other stews. Even if you aren't from around here (don't mean to rub it in), you can probably find something similar in your grocery store's freezer section.

Frozen Vegetables for Main Dishes

These days you can get all sorts of single vegetables and vegetable blends in freezer bags. My staples include broccoli, cauliflower, carrots, bok choi, spinach, kale and other greens, and different "ethnic" blends like stir-fry, southwest, Tex-Mex, and Italian. If the bag includes a sauce packet, throw it in the garbage before you start cooking. It will be full of sugar, oil, salt, and probably artificial ingredients as well.

Daily Trips

My daily grocery trips are typically a tiny version of "makin' groceries," meant to top up anything that I'm out of, or to satisfy my *envie* (pronounced "on-vee"; bayou-speak for "craving").

I don't use a shopping cart. Instead, I grab a small basket, and when it's full, I'm done shopping. That way I don't shop opportunistically and avoid the temptation to stock up on sale items that I don't need or want.

An example of a daily shop might look like this: a bag of kale, a few potatoes, and 3-4 apples. That on top of the frozen veggies and precooked grain I already have at home will get me through supper tonight, breakfast tomorrow, and maybe lunch tomorrow.

This way of shopping is not only much more calorically dilute than the way I used to do it, but it's also lighter on the wallet and better for the environment. I'm eating lower on the food chain, so there are fewer middlemen and less packaging.

On these daily trips, I often get (or at least feel) hungry. Something about being in the presence of food makes me want to eat. If you ever find yourself craving a bite while you're food shopping, you know what I mean. So I often also get something I can eat right away, as soon as I leave the store.

This might be a single loose carrot (as opposed to a pound or 5-pound bag), an apple, or a tub of precut pineapple or watermelon. If I'm feeling particularly virtuous, I'll go for a bag of fresh cut cauliflower and broccoli. I think of this as a practice of delaying immediate gratification in pursuit of long-term goals, because it's obvious that a piece of raw broccoli is not nearly as tasty as fried or baked chips, even the ones in the "health food" aisle.

My stomach stretch receptors are satisfied even though I don't get the dopamine fireworks in my brain that I used to associate with eating. You'll be surprised at how quickly you will adapt and feel satisfied without those fireworks, and how empowered you become – in all areas of your life that require self-discipline – by developing the habit of choosing healthy over hyperpalatable.

Sometimes, if I'm looking for a slightly richer snack, I'll eat a few walnuts. Nuts are healthy in small quantities, but as we saw in the NAQ chapter, they can be problematic for overweight people as they're so calorically dense.

If you do choose to include some nuts in your diet, please forget about buying in bulk. Avoid those giant, resealable bags of nuts. I know the nutrition facts on the bag says that it's 48 servings, but that's not how fat people think. A bag is a serving, no matter how big, and we eat until it's empty.

Again, think in terms of NAQ. A giant bag of shelled nuts every week is a stupendously UNnatural quantity.

I have two shopping tricks for limiting the amount of nuts I consume. One is to buy a small bag of nuts from the baking section, rather than from the snacks aisle. The baking section has nuts in quantities meant for recipes, rather than direct snacking.

The second trick you can use only if your store has a bulk section, like those found in many health food and natural stores (like Whole Foods). Grab a scant ⅓ of a scoop — a single snack serving — to guarantee that you aren't stockpiling. And be clear on what you're buying them for: if you want a handful in your smoothie bowl tomorrow morning, then make sure you don't eat the entire bag in your vehicle on the way home.

While I have a problem buying nuts in bulk, I know Howard doesn't. He keeps them handy in the freezer, and saves money by buying in bulk. The meta-lesson here is to know yourself. And the best way to do that, as we've said a bunch of times in other chapters, is by experimenting, treating every failure as useful data, and trying something else next time.

Extreme Shopping

It's pretty easy to eat well when you have grocery stores and supermarkets at your disposal, once you master the routines and tricks that keep you focused on whole, unprocessed plants and away from the animal products and processed junk. Where people get hung up is when there's "nothing healthy to eat": when you're hungry and the only place to get grub is somewhere like a convenience store, gas station, airport, or sports stadium.

My businesses (owning and running pump stations and a trailer park) keep me hopping around and on the road a lot around my South Louisiana parish. Convenience stores used to be my downfall. I would drool over the sad pizza slices that had spent all day under the warming lights, the chicken gizzards, the boudin balls (Cajun sausage filling that has been balled up, battered, and deep fried). Since I'm often on the road for hours, far from grocery stores, I had to figure out other ways to make sure I was eating reasonably healthy food.

One strategy is to always be prepared. Keep some healthy stuff with you at all times. Pack healthy meals and snacks before you leave in the morning.

That's fine — it's never a bad idea to be prepared. But you also shouldn't rely on preparation exclusively, because it makes us fragile when we don't prepare. People throw this excuse at me all the time: "Man, meal prep is my downfall. I don't have time to prep, and if I don't prep, then I fail."

I don't have time to prep either. I'm too busy living my life, and I'm not a planner by nature. Maybe I could force myself. But the point I want to make is that it's not necessary.

Preparation is NOT a prerequisite to success in healthy eating. The trick is to make good choices no matter what life throws your way. There's always a better option than the ones that led to the overweight or unhealthy body you're trying to change.

OK, you're not going to make a gourmet NAQ meal from a convenience store. And you won't find cut broccoli or even, often, a piece of fruit. But even at a bait and tackle shop on the bayou, miles from anywhere, you can still make the best of it.

These types of stores typically sell snack packs of nuts. Make sure the ones you get have no added oil, so avoid the Planters' Deluxe mixes and Colossal Cashews and the like, filled with sugar and extra fat and artificial flavorings. Stick to raw almonds or walnuts if possible, or find regular roasted nuts (often they're labeled "natural"). If you're lucky, you can find a bag of in-shell peanuts.

Sometimes I'll grab a pickle if they have a vat. And I always get a big plastic gallon jug of water. That much liquid helps fill you up, keeps you hydrated, and is for some reason cheaper than a liter of Dasani or some other fancy-sounding brand.

I'm not telling you to make a life out of pickles and roasted almonds, but they're acceptable options when you have no better choice, and when you're eating them in such small quantities and so rarely that they're immaterial to your overall health trajectory.

When those "emergency foods" are drowned out by the bulk of what you keep your house stocked with, then the damage they do is so minimal that it doesn't really matter. They're what Brooke Goldner, MD, calls a "paper cut" food choice.

And remember that while the goal is always 100% perfection, be wary of using that goal as an excuse to give up and make terrible choices if perfection isn't possible in a given situation. Rather, we're trying to be what Joel Fuhrman, MD, calls "Nutritarians": people who make the best available nutritional choice under every circumstance.

How to Transition

Howard here, to talk with you about how to get from Point A (where you are now) to Point B (your ideal way of eating). The first thing to know is that Point B is probably going to change over time. And that's a good thing.

When I began my own transition, there were a whole bunch of foods I was certain I would never ever give up. Buttered corn. Pesto pasta with fresh parmesan. Pepe's Pizza (if you've ever lived in New Haven, Connecticut, you know what I'm talking about).

But over time, my Point B has shifted. Some foods just lost their appeal as my taste buds changed. Some foods still taste good, but make me feel terrible after I eat them. Some foods still call to me, but I value my long-term well-being and athletic prowess more than a Levain's chocolate chip cookie, though it's a great dopamine rush (New York's Upper West Siders, do you feel me?).

So hold your Point B lightly, and be willing to adjust and adapt as you go. Once you attain the results you were looking for originally, you're a new, different person. That new person probably wants bigger and better results in their life.

And as Josh is so fond of repeating, Results Dictate Sufficiency. If you want bigger and better results, then you're going to have to up your game: Menu, Movement, and Mindset should all evolve and grow to support your higher aspirations.

Transition styles

The second thing to consider is how you like to approach the process of change.

There are as many different successful transitions to NAQ eating as there are transitioners. What works for you, works for you. That said, I'd like to highlight three basic patterns. Chances are one of them will make the most sense to you. Start there, as it's the one you're most likely to stick with.

Transition Style #1: Overnight

Some people transition all at once. From the outside, this can look as if the person just woke up one morning a completely different person.

I've seen people undergo transitions like this after visiting a farm sanctuary or watching a powerful documentary. Several folks I know changed instantaneously after a massive health scare, like a near-fatal stroke or heart attack. And more than one person I've worked with has adopted a strict plant-based diet after a consultation with a charismatic powerhouse like Caldwell Esselstyn, MD.

The overnight transition, when successful, usually occurs as a logical outgrowth of a complete inner transformation: what behavior scientist BJ Fogg calls an epiphany. The new you simply can't eat the food that the old you found just fine. Because of new information, or a new frame of reference, your eating habits and other behaviors must shift for you to remain a congruent human being.

If you have such an epiphany, then go with the flow. Purge your kitchen, either into garbage bags or into boxes destined for a food pantry. Reread the first part of this chapter and head to the grocery store, shopping list in hand.

Choose a couple of staple meals, and get clear on the benefits of keeping things really simple as your skills and capabilities catch up to your intentions. Be careful that you don't rush things out of a sense of urgency. You don't want to experience blowback from attempting more than your current food prep ability can support.

Transition Style #2: Gradual

Many people instead transition gradually, over time. Two steps forward and one step back. Weeks of progress followed by lapses, binges, loosened rules and then recommitment.

Gradual transition can be highly effective, but it can also be crazy-making. You can find yourself eating foods that you no longer approve of, which can generate all kinds of guilt and shame and self-doubt.

The key to a successful gradual transition is to keep your eye on consistent progress. The important thing is to DO. The pace you choose is far less important than the experience of leaning into progress every day.

Don't let your fear of thrashing around without knowing what you're doing keep you from DOing. Even if it's wrong, DO. The more you DO, the faster you learn what not to do, and the best ways to move forward.

If you're a "gradualizer," embrace both the end goal and the journey. Savor each advance you make, and strive to consolidate your gains so that you aren't yo-yoing back and forth between better and worse.

Avoid this yo-yoing by keeping things simple, and getting greedy for feedback. If you make 10 NAQ meals and hate nine of them, you've just found one meal that you can make again and again. A measly 10% success rate puts you ahead of the game, if you pay attention to what works and keep building upon it. After all, you never have to make the bad meals again, while you can add the good ones to your growing food repertoire.

Start today by making one simple NAQ meal. Have an oatmeal bowl for breakfast instead of eggs, bacon, and waffles. Leave the chicken strips and oil out of tonight's stir-fry. Get a can of beans and mix in a can of corn and half a cup of salsa, and serve over steamed greens, instead of picking up a burrito from your local chain Tex-Mex joint.

Transition Style #3: Tectonic

The tectonic style gets its name from the way the earth's plates move: whole regions shift at once, and then gradually, everything above ground settles into its new configuration.

I find the tectonic approach to be the most effective for most people. It combines the best of the overnight and the gradual: it gives you a strong sense of forward progress, while allowing your inner self and your outer behaviors to stay in close alignment.

When you go tectonic, you upgrade a whole category rather than an individual food or habit.

The classic tectonic first move is to adopt a single NAQ breakfast as your daily default. For me, that was a green smoothie with fruit. (Other tectonic breakfasts: cooked oatmeal, muesli with fruit; a raw oats bowl with mashed bananas and fruit.)

With a single change, I upgraded roughly one-third of my meals and calories from health-compromising to health-promoting.

The key to tectonic transition is not to aim for immediate perfection in all areas, but rather to make a significant change that you can maintain as a beachhead to serve as a defensible position as you prepare for the next change. You stick to this one simple yet significant shift until it becomes normal and natural. And then add another tectonic shift.

As long as each change is for the better, you're going to make predictable and meaningful progress.

Another tectonic strategy is to shorten your "feeding window": the hours between which you take in calories during the day. Lots of us have struggled with late-night snacking that can undo an entire day's worth of virtuous eating. If you make the tectonic shift to eating from 8am until 7pm, and then fasting for 13 hours each night, you'll probably lose weight and feel better even if you don't improve the quality of your Menu at first.

A third tectonic strategy is to eliminate or promote an entire class of foods. The ultimate tectonic elimination is dairy (aka the baby food meant for a different species). All you have to do is think about it rationally for a minute: milk and cheese are staples of the Western diet, but enslaving billions of animals so we can steal their infants' food source is a pretty perverse thing when you remove the cultural blinders that make it seem OK.

Eliminating dairy is actually really easy, thanks to the dozens of plant-based dairy alternatives that can replace milk, butter, yogurt, and even cheese. Which brings me to the issue of transitional foods.

Transitional foods

I think transitional foods are great. From plant-based cheeses to nut milks to low-fat vegan desserts to ultra-realistic hamburgers made from soy and pea protein, these foods can play a really useful role in helping wean you off addictive and harmful foods.

The problem comes when the transition foods become the new normal, and you stop there. You wouldn't book a flight from New York to Los Angeles and decide to stop traveling when your plane stops to refuel in Detroit.

Vegan junk food won't solve our health problems. Just because it's less terrible than the Standard Western Diet doesn't mean it's going to change your weight or your health trajectory. According to Kim Williams, MD, past president of the American College of Cardiology, junk food that's high in trans fat, whether vegan or not, is worse for your health than meat.

If you choose to use these transitional foods as a wedge between you and your old favorites, make sure you have a plan to continue your journey to your desired destination. The sooner you phase out the junk, the sooner your taste buds will get used to the flavors and textures of the real foods that humans evolved to eat.

And the sooner you'll start attaining the results and life you want.

Transition Tools

After you've been at this for a while, you'll acquire the knack of eating according to NAQ. In the beginning, you want to keep it simple. Focus on the single strategy, single visual cue, and single skill below.

Strategy: Stock Up on Default Foods

The most powerful strategy by far for eating healthier is strict simplicity in your food choices. Eat the same breakfast, lunch, and dinner every day for a month. Then add a second kind of dinner. Then a third. When you feel like a pro, add a second lunch, too.

Once you've chosen your defaults, make sure you always have the ingredients on hand. If your dinner thing is rice and beans over veggies, buy bags of rice, cans of beans, and bags of frozen veggies. Stock your pantry with these three items. Keep several jars of salsa (or whatever condiment you choose) in reserve so you have no excuse to stray.

Also, limit the variety of ingredients to keep things simple. The fewer different kinds of ingredients in your pantry and refrigerator, the easier it is to decide what meals to prepare, and the sooner you'll move from thinking to DOing.

Visual Cue: Eat the Rainbow

The single key visual cue for healthier eating is the rainbow. As we've seen, the more colors of produce on your plate, and the brighter those colors are, the healthier your meal.

If you make a collage out of every day's food, you should see a beautiful palate of rich, vibrant, delicious, colors.

Skill: Label Reading

For many of us, the thing that trips up our attempts at healthier eating is sneaky unhealthy ingredients in processed foods.

Whether it's tons of sugar disguised by a pseudonym (natural sweetener, corn syrup, dextrose, barley malt, ethyl maltol, cane juice crystals, and Sucanat, to name just a few), sneaky dairy (whey, casein, ghee, lactose), artificial ingredients (you know, the ones you can't pronounce), boatloads of fat, or an unconscionable amount of salt, food companies will do whatever it takes to keep you hooked.

That's why label reading is key. Here's a guide to reading labels like a pro, so you can keep the crap off your plate and out of your belly.

Label Literacy

The main ingredients in a natural and optimal human diet typically don't come with labels: fruits, vegetables, nuts and seeds, legumes, and whole grains. So as long as you aren't living on things that come from cans and boxes, you don't have to worry too much about reading food labels.

Sometimes, though, you may want to spice up your main ingredients with prepared sauces, spices, condiments, and plant foods that have been processed to some extent—so you need to know a few things about reading labels.

Skill #1: Knowing what to ignore

Rule 1: Ignore all claims on the front of the package.

The frozen dessert calling you from the supermarket freezer case may be GMO-free, gluten-free, lactose-free, low glycemic, and contain protein and fiber, but it's probably still crap.

Rule 2: Ignore all claims not on the nutrition label or ingredients list.

They're just marketing, and are often misleading or irrelevant.

Rule 3: Ignore most of what's on the nutrition label.

Politicians, lobbyists, and scientists spend a lot of time arguing about what should go on food labels, and industry hacks and some scientists promote the inclusion of as many known nutrients as possible.

But that's a terrible idea, for several reasons.

First, there's no clear connection in the research between any specific nutrient and any desirable or undesirable health outcome.

Second, listing nutrients misleads the public into thinking that we should be counting and measuring these things.

Third, it leads the public to believe that any nutrient not on the list is not important.

Fourth, it encourages processed food manufacturers to "fortify" their products with nutrient powders or slurries so they can tout them as nutritious, when many studies have shown that supplemental nutrients (such as those consumed as pills or in fortified foods) do little good, and can do considerable harm.

When reading labels, ignore the amounts of vitamin A, riboflavin, iron, and so on. Your job is to get all that good stuff from whole foods in their natural state.

Your main job as a label reader is to look for the bad stuff—so you can keep it out of your cart, off your shelf, away from your plate, and far away from your body.

Skill #2: Deciphering Hidden Ingredients

Ingredients are listed in descending order of weight. That is, the first ingredient comprises the highest percentage of weight of the total product, and so on down the line.

Here's the ingredient list for a popular brand of salsa verde: fresh tomatillos, green chili, water, onions, fresh jalapeños, salt, spices.

Assuming you know what tomatillos and jalapeños are (vegetables common in Central American cuisine), everything here looks perfectly normal. A bunch of plants, water, salt, and spices. No problems, right?

Hang on a second.

What are "spices"?

Huh? We all know what spices are, right? Cumin, coriander, cinnamon, curry, MSG, oregano, marjoram...

Wait—MSG? Monosodium glutamate?

Yup, that nasty flavor-enhancing chemical, which can cause headaches, muscle aches, fatigue, and a whole host of other symptoms, can legally hide behind the innocuous word "spices."

Another hidden minefield word in ingredient lists is "flavoring." When you see "natural flavorings," you probably imagine harmless essences of vanilla and almond.

But the truth is, "natural flavorings" on a label could mean pretty much anything. Flavor enhancers (yes, another chance for our old nemesis MSG to sneak back onto the Menu), synthetic flavors constructed in test tubes and containing just a few molecules of anything nature produced—the sky's the limit. One common ingredient to give desserts a vanilla flavor – and I am not making this up – is beaver butt extract. Don't believe me? Google "castoreum safety" and follow the top link to a National Institutes of Health abstract of a scientific paper on the safety of these glandular secretions in food.

Discovering Hidden Sugar

Next time you're in the store, take a look at the ingredients list for Hershey's chocolate syrup.

Sorry, I mean "Hershey's Genuine Chocolate Flavor Syrup." They're technically not allowed to call it chocolate, because, well, it doesn't actually contain enough cocoa to be so named.

High fructose corn syrup (HFCS), the first ingredient, has become pretty well known in the past few years, thanks to various folks pointing out that the stuff is everywhere, heavily subsidized by the US government, and at least as bad for us as sugar (and probably worse).

Now, just in case you're thinking, "Gee, if the first ingredient is basically sugar, this stuff must be plenty sweet," you should realize that there are actually two *more* sweeteners included on the ingredient list: "corn syrup" (second item, just after HFCS), and sugar itself.

Perhaps Hershey's thought that caring moms wouldn't like to see sugar as the main ingredient, so they put their scientists and marketers on the problem.

Watching Out for Other Additives

Let's also take a look at some of the ingredients that follow sugar: potassium sorbate, mono- and diglycerides, polysorbate 60, and artificial flavor.

I don't want to get into the purposes, chemical makeup, and health effects of these products here. Most of the thousands of food additives are untested, and there's virtually no research into how they interact with each other to wreak havoc in our bodies. We are basically an uncontrolled experiment carried out by the food industry.

Follow the "grandmother rule": if you can't pronounce it, don't eat it.

If you can't trace it back to something in nature, don't eat it. If you can't make it without beakers, test tubes, and Bunsen burners, don't eat it.

Identifying animal ingredients

You should also keep an eye out for the sneaky ways that food companies hide animal products in their ingredient lists. If you see whey, casein, caseinate, sodium caseinate, gelatin, lactose, lecithin (from eggs, if it doesn't specifically say "soy" or "sunflower"), rennet, monoglycerides, or glycerides, you're looking at animal products in your food.

Skill #3: Doing the math on serving size, fat, fiber, and salt

Let's head back to the nutritional label for the third big skill: doing the math. The nutrient amounts listed on the label are "per serving." Just how big is a serving?

Sneaky Serving Sizes

To find out what the manufacturer means by a serving, you have to check out the label's Serving Size and Servings Per Container information.

For example, one serving of Hershey's chocolate flavored syrup consists of 1 tablespoon of syrup. For most hot sauces, a single serving is one teaspoon.

Why is serving size so important? Because the important information on the nutrition label is per single serving, so many manufacturers try to get serving sizes as small as possible to make their food seem less bad than it is.

For example, there are just 160 calories in a serving of Oreo cookies. But a serving is defined as three cookies.

I don't know about you, but when I was eating Oreos, a serving was more like an entire sleeve - or box.

My point is, if you're consuming thousands of calories of a product but reading the label as if you were eating fewer than 200, you'll vastly underestimate the impact of that consumption on your caloric budget and your health.

% Calories from Fat

Once you know the serving size, you can calculate the amount of fat a particular food is adding to your diet.

Depending on your metabolism and lifestyle, you'll want to limit overall fat intake to 10–20% of calories over the course of a given day or week. When you exceed 20% of calories from fat, you will be driven to overeat since high fat foods are calorically dense (recall the almost empty third stomach from the image earlier in this chapter). As we've seen, the NAQ foods tend to be calorically dilute, whereas the high-calorie foods (which get that way because they're high in fat) are rarely dilute.

If you eat mostly processed foods with added oils, you'll find it almost impossible to stay below the 20% mark. And if weight loss is a current goal, then 10-15% is a much better range to aim for.

Unfortunately, nowhere on the nutrition label are we told this percentage—or any of the other percentages we discuss below —directly.

We have to figure them out. It's easy at the moment, but new FDA nutritional label regulations will make it trickier in the future. The new labels are being phased in now, and will be required by January 1, 2020 for companies with over $10 million in annual sales, and January 1, 2021, for smaller companies.

The Current Label

First, find the total calories per serving size. In Oreos, it's 160. Now look for calories from fat: 60.

Time for a little arithmetic.

The percentage of calories from fat is 60/160, or 37.5%.

As you can see, the Oreos contain about 2 to 4 times the fat than you can get from eating a NAQ diet.

Now, some whole plant foods do provide more than 10% of their calories from fat. An average avocado, for example, is about 80% fat.

But avocados are whole plant foods, and they also contain water, fiber, and more nutrients than science will ever be able to discover and name. I also don't recommend an all-avocado diet.

The important thing isn't the ratio for each item you eat; it's the overall ratio in your diet.

The New Label

As you can see, in the new nutrition facts label (the one on the right), the "calories from fat" line item is gone. That means, to find out the percentage of calories from fat, you've got to add a second step: calculating calories from fat.

Nutrition Facts

Serving Size 2/3 cup (55g)
Servings Per Container About 8

Amount Per Serving

Calories 230	Calories from Fat 72
	% Daily Value*
Total Fat 8g	**12%**
Saturated Fat 1g	**5%**
Trans Fat 0g	
Cholesterol 0mg	**0%**
Sodium 160mg	**7%**
Total Carbohydrate 37g	**12%**
Dietary Fiber 4g	**16%**
Sugars 1g	
Protein 3g	
Vitamin A	10%
Vitamin C	8%
Calcium	20%
Iron	45%

* Percent Daily Values are based on a 2,000 calorie diet. Your daily value may be higher or lower depending on your calorie needs.

	Calories:	2,000	2,500
Total Fat	Less than	65g	80g
Sat Fat	Less than	20g	25g
Cholesterol	Less than	300mg	300mg
Sodium	Less than	2,400mg	2,400mg
Total Carbohydrate		300g	375g
Dietary Fiber		25g	30g

Nutrition Facts

8 servings per container
Serving size   2/3 cup (55g)

Amount per serving

Calories   230

	% Daily Value*
Total Fat 8g	**10%**
Saturated Fat 1g	**5%**
Trans Fat 0g	
Cholesterol 0mg	**0%**
Sodium 160mg	**7%**
Total Carbohydrate 37g	**13%**
Dietary Fiber 4g	**14%**
Total Sugars 12g	
Includes 10g Added Sugars	**20%**
Protein 3g	
Vitamin D 2mcg	10%
Calcium 260mg	20%
Iron 8mg	45%
Potassium 235mg	6%

* The % Daily Value (DV) tells you how much a nutrient in a serving of food contributes to a daily diet. 2,000 calories a day is used for general nutrition advice.

Look for the Total Fat line item.

In the example shown, that's 8g, or 8 grams.

There are 9 calories in every gram of fat. So in this case, multiply 8 (the number of grams of fat) x 9 (the number of calories per gram of fat) to get a total of 72 calories from fat per serving.

Now you can perform the previous calculation to get the percentage of calories from fat, dividing 72 calories from fat by the total of 230 calories per serving: 72/230, or 31.3% of calories from fat.

Carbohydrates to Fiber Ratio

Another important metric that helps us avoid highly processed foods is the carbohydrate-to-fiber ratio.

In nature, there are very few foods with lots of carbohydrates and very little fiber. In fact, the only one I can think of is honey.

So when you see a label on a packaged food that lists lots of carbohydrates and very little fiber, you know that the food has been processed to remove that fiber and just give you calories that get digested way too quickly.

Dr. Michael Greger of NutritionFacts.org recommends a carbohydrate-to-fiber ratio of no more than 5:1. In the above label, we can see 37 grams of total carbohydrate, and just 4 grams of fiber. 37/4 = 9.25.

9.25 is greater than 5, which disqualifies this food. It's too processed, with too much fiber stripped away, and too many "empty" carbohydrates from sugar and white flour.

Salt Content

The rule of thumb here is *no more sodium than calories*. That is, if you consume 2000 calories per day, you should limit your daily intake of sodium to 2000 milligrams (mg).

So for any food with a label, the ratio of sodium milligrams to calories should be no greater than 1.

For example, some white bread has 240 mg sodium per 110 calories, or 2.4 times as much sodium as calories. So this food is a sodium no-no.

The Condiment Exception

You don't have to worry about the percentage of fat in a food that you're eating only in tiny amounts. For example, soy sauce is really high in sodium, which would be a giant problem if you were drinking it from Big Gulps. If, instead, you're flavoring a stir-fry with a teaspoon, the extra sodium gets diluted by all the extremely-low-sodium vegetables and brown rice.

Likewise, if you find a brand of hummus that has 25% of fat from calories and you spread a half tablespoon onto a veggie wrap, I hereby declare that hummus a condiment. If, on the other hand, you're shoveling heaping spoonfuls into your mouth, that hummus has graduated from condiment to full-on food, and needs to be treated accordingly.

I still wouldn't let my condiments contain artificial ingredients, but you can loosen the guidelines on fat percentage, carbohydrate-to-fiber ratio, and sodium-to-calorie ratio.

The Bottom Line on Reading Food Labels

1. Ignore most of the information on the label. It's not important.
2. Reject unpronounceable and "sneaky" ingredients.
3. Check the serving size so you know how many calories and nutrients you're *really* eating.
4. Reject foods that get more than 20% of their calories from fat.
5. Reject foods with a carbohydrate-to-fiber ratio greater than 5:1.
6. Reject foods with more milligrams of sodium than calories per serving.
7. The exception to rules 4-6: condiments with very few calories that you eat in tiny amounts.
8. Remember, foods that come from cans, boxes, and jars are your condiments and extras. The basis of a healthy diet is plants, as close to their natural state as possible.

Important Perspective: It's Bigger Than the Scale

Before we leave the Menu part of this book, I want to emphasize that our focus on eating wholesome, calorically dilute food is not simply about how many pounds you weigh.

Most of us have been on diets before (for some of us, dozens, and for pretty much all of our adult lives). We're all good at changing what we put on our plates and in our mouths in order to manipulate the number on a scale.

But none of us have ever found that a sustainable practice. Once we hit our magic number, we're not prepared to sustain it. In fact, seeing the scale tell us that we've "won" is often a trigger to celebrate. And we celebrate by going off the diet that got us there in the first place.

While the scale is useful as a point of feedback to make sure we're on the right track and DOing at the right intensity, it's not the ultimate measure of success. If you make these eating changes, you'll almost definitely lose weight. But you'll also gain something much more important; something so important, in fact, that you'll come to think of the weight loss as a nice little side effect rather than the point.

The dirty little secret of Big Change is that the minute we think we've achieved the big change and we're done, we're actually just starting.

Now that our body and lifestyle habits are in order, we can start living like the authentic human we've always been.

Now we can start dreaming, imagining, visualizing, and DOing, and approach the *real* Big Changes that happen when we're living a life in harmony with nature and our highest selves.

Dr Greger's Black Box Warning

When we showed this chapter to Michael Greger, MD, of NutritionFacts.org, he requested that we include a warning about vitamin B_{12}.

You see, if you end up transitioning all the way to a mostly or completely plant-based diet, you'll want to supplement with B_{12}.

And when a lot of people hear that, they start thinking, "Well then, doesn't that mean that a plant-based diet isn't natural, since I'd need to supplement?"

So here's the scoop:

B_{12} doesn't come from plants or animals; instead, it's made by bacteria. In the olden days, we got plenty of B_{12} just from eating our veggies (or working on farms). These days, with chlorinated water, sterile soil, and national fear of dirt, B_{12} is hard to come by in our natural environment.

The only place those bacteria can still thrive is in the guts of animals like cows, chickens, goats, and so on. So if you stop consuming animals, you're at risk of developing a B_{12} deficiency over time. Even if you tend an organic garden, you should still supplement.

Here's Dr G's recommendation: "The cheapest way to get our B_{12} is probably one 2500 microgram sublingual, chewable, or liquid supplement of cyanocobalamin once a week. This stuff is dirt cheap. You can find a twenty-year supply online for 40 bucks. All the B_{12} our body needs for $2 a year! Of course, the stuff doesn't last twenty years. It has a four-year expiration date, so share it with some friends."

MOVEMENT

We put Menu first because food is utterly fundamental to our body's survival. If we're not fueling ourselves properly, it's really, really hard to sustain a daily practice of Movement. And it's darn near impossible to have a positive Mindset when our brain is dealing with a chronically overfed and malnourished body.

But Movement is a close second in terms of ultimate importance. And as we've seen, Movement and Menu are closely connected. Just as when you get Menu wrong, it's almost impossible to generate Movement over time, if you get it wrong, it's hard to sustain your Menu resolve when cravings hit.

Still, Movement alone can be a great place to start.

Josh lost over 100 pounds just from joining a gym, working out religiously, and self-identifying as a runner, without really addressing the food issue much at all.

So wherever you are in your journey and whatever you focus on first, you can make progress that will get you to the next level of fitness and health. If the last chapter overwhelmed you, or if you're still under the spell of paleo "Bro Science" or terrified of lectins or some other BS (sorry, but science is science), you can definitely begin here.

We'll check out what we're up against: the evolutionary forces that conspire to keep us on the couch, and a modern environment that accommodates and amplifies those forces. We'll see what it means to take our MED (Minimum Exertion Demanded) in that modern environment, and why it's still crucial for our physical and psychological wellbeing.

We'll examine the three qualities of natural human Movement: functional, challenging, and wholistic.

Then we'll spend a lot of time helping you get started, with strategies and tactics and hacks designed to get you walking or jogging or running or swimming or whatever, and helping you learn how to push yourself and persist without ending up on crutches or pain meds.

Finally, we'll examine some of the mental aspects of Movement, so you can overcome that evolutionary laziness when it rears its ugly and predictable head those cold, wet mornings when you just don't want to get out of bed.

Why Effortful Movement is Hard

Human physiology and psychology evolved in an environment where Movement was necessary much of the time. Whether hunting or gathering, collecting firewood and building materials, or migrating toward water and game and fruit and away from bad weather, humans were basically on our feet, straining our muscles and burning calories, just about all the time.

To ensure our survival, we developed a bias toward rest. Whenever we didn't need to be exerting ourselves, we rested. We recovered. We conserved our precious energy because we never knew when we'd have to spend it foraging for our lunch or avoiding becoming some other creature's lunch. In other words, we'd always choose rest when it was naturally attainable.

Now, of course, this impulse toward rest and recovery is totally accommodated by our environment.

As we saw in chapter 5, we can cover hundreds of miles a day while sitting on our asses, propelled by the remains of dead dinosaurs through the alchemy of fossil fuels.

We can shop for food on motorized carts at Walmart, or online at Amazon. We get our cooking and heating fuel delivered straight to our homes via tanker or power line. We pick up wall studs and decking in our pickup trucks.

We can replace just about every muscular exertion imaginable with a motor or with someone else's labor.

And still our psychology warns us against doing any more physical activity than absolutely necessary, just in case we encounter a challenge that requires all our capacity to overcome.

So the heart of Movement is a conscious decision to override this biological programming, and move voluntarily the way our environment used to force us to move.

Now that we're clear on the attitude we need, let's look at what natural human Movement—the kind of Movement we aim to recreate and pay homage to—is like. And once again, we're going to turn to our evolutionary heritage for clues to how we were designed to move.

Natural Human Movement

There are a million books on exercise, and the last thing you need is another one. So we're going to avoid the entire concept of exercise, which implies that moving is a "thing" that we can either add on to our daily routine or not. Rather, we're going to talk about Movement.

Up until recently in human development, Movement was life. If you were alive, you were moving. When you stopped moving, due to injury, infirmity, or disease, you died. There were no ICUs to keep you alive or motorized vehicles to allow you to pursue your NAQ of food. Don't get us wrong; we're happy to be living in our modern world. We just don't want these technological advances to compromise our health and happiness – and they don't have to!

So as we go about revising our lives to honor the MED we've evolved for, what do we know about the varieties, frequencies, and intensities of Movement that are most fitting for human beings?

Long walks? High intensity interval training? Many repetitions of light weights? Short sets of extremely heavy weights?

Every day, it seems, there's a new study on exercise that contradicts all the previous studies.

So instead of jumping from finding to finding (most of which come from short-term studies in artificial laboratory conditions and squinting at individual variables rather than looking at the big picture for an answer), we're going to ground ourselves in common sense.

What are our bodies designed to DO, and what were they asked to DO by the environment in which they evolved? It turns out there are three criteria for a healthy human Movement protocol:

1. It is based on Movements that were functional in our ancestral environment.
2. It is physically challenging, and alternates between stress and recovery.
3. It involves moving the entire body as a whole, rather than isolating certain muscles and ranges of motion.

Human Movement is Functional in Our Ancestral Environment

Like every other organism, we evolved our current form in a tight match with our environment. Just as giraffes evolved long necks to outcompete other land animals in their ability to munch on the leaves of tall trees, we evolved our unique structures and abilities to fit in our own ecological niche.

Every species that survives does so because it has its niche. And that niche determines the Movement best suited to gathering resources necessary for survival and reproduction within it.

Birds fly. Fish swim. Kangaroos hop. Snakes slither.

And humans? What distinguishes humans from other animals? And more specifically from our nearest relatives, the other great apes like gorillas and chimpanzees?

The big thing, the one honkingly obvious difference, is the way we move upon the earth. We walk upright, on two legs, and can do so at a pretty quick clip for a really long time. We are the beasts who can run for hours.

Human Movement is Bipedal Locomotion

This upright gait is known by eggheads as bipedal ("two-legged") locomotion ("moving from place to place"). Since we want to sound smart and sophisticated, we'll use that phrase as well.

Once we evolved the ability to walk and run on two legs without needing our hands and arms for balance, everything changed. We could now collect fruits, leafy green vegetables, and tubers with our freed-up hands. We could use our manual dexterity to create baskets, tools, and weapons that made us super-hunter-gatherers.

We could carry our offspring, or manufacture carriers to keep them on our bodies while we walked. We could then give birth to smaller, more helpless babies, since we could carry and protect them for longer periods of time. Giving birth to tinier babies meant female humans could have smaller hips. This allowed them even greater efficiency in walking and running.

And all the rest followed—bigger brains, the advantages of social collaboration and the development of symbolic language, persistence hunting, the discovery of agriculture, the rise of industrial society, and the digital age.

The base of the pyramid of human physiology, culture, and accomplishment is bipedal locomotion.

We used it to survive and to reproduce until we became the dominant species on the planet. We gathered food while walking. We sprinted away from predators, and banded together to fight against them. We organized hunting parties and preyed on animals who could run two to three times as fast as us, by using the "slow and steady" approach and tiring them to the point of collapse.

We migrated over tens of thousands of miles, populating the entire earth.

And on a daily basis, we walked our territory, surveying its resources and threats and marking its boundaries as a warning to potential competitors, human and otherwise.

Running, jogging, hiking, walking — these are the Movement patterns that made us human, and make us human even today.

Baby, You Were Born to Run

You can find proof of our natural affinity with bipedal locomotion not just in our evolutionary past, but in our current biology. Unlike just about every other animal, humans can sweat. Which means we can dissipate heat more quickly and efficiently than any animal we might be chasing over a long distance.

Your dog might pull you on a 3-mile jog through the neighborhood, but Spot isn't going to run a marathon, ever. It would be animal abuse to try to drag him 26.2 miles. He's just not built for it. But we are.

Our feet are designed to cover all different kinds of terrain. Our hips allow for efficient leg swinging with minimal energy expenditure.

If you don't believe us, do yourself a favor and spend some time at the finish line of a marathon. You'll see all kinds of bodies — long and short, lean and stout, muscular and skinny, soft and overweight, sighted and blind, hearing and Deaf, old and young, male and female — crossing that 26.2 mark with smiles and tears on their faces and fists in the air.

It's a human thing.

If you want a lot more information on the human physiological adaptations to bipedal locomotion, check out Christopher

McDougall's epic book, *Born to Run*. It was one of the major influences on Josh's decision to take running seriously.

Cheap and Easy

Starting to "exercise" usually involves buying gear, joining a gym, or getting new clothes.

That's no accident, of course. The media messages about exercise are paid for by an industry that wants you to spend money. And there's absolutely nothing wrong with gear, memberships, or cool and functional clothes. We both have plenty of all of these things.

But bipedal locomotion doesn't *require* any expenditure at all. You already own clothes and footwear. You can walk just about anywhere. All that's required to get into this form of Movement is to get up off the couch and start moving!

Movement is Brain Food

Not only is bipedal locomotion good for the body, it's also good for the brain and the mood.

Any form of exercise triggers the production and release of a protein called BDNF, which is short for brain-derived neurotrophic factor. Long story short, BDNF allows our brains to make new cells and to take in new information.

If you think about it, it makes a ton of sense that our brains would be buzzed into hyper learning during Movement. One of our main biological imperatives is conservation: of calories, of Movement, of everything potentially scarce in our environment. Our brains are total energy hogs; at just about 3% of our body weight, those mushy cauliflowers between our ears use up around 25% of our total caloric intake.

That's why we can go into "eat anything within reach" mode when our blood sugar drops. Our brain signals "Emergency, emergency" and convinces us that everything is fair game, whether it's on our food plan or not.

Because the brain uses up that much energy, our conservation imperative means we would have evolved to keep it turned down to basic life support unless we required a heavy dose of learning.

When we're sitting down by our hut, we typically don't need to learn anything. But when we're out and about, stumbling upon fields of yams or meadows with fruit-bearing trees, encountering wild animals, potable streams and unpredictable weather patterns, learning and problem solving and laying down new memories are really good ideas.

In other words, it makes sense that the act of Movement would trigger the production of BDNF, because it meant we could use our big brains to our best advantage as we covered our territory.

Movement is also a powerful mood enhancer, triggering the same cascade of happy juice chemicals like dopamine, serotonin, and oxytocin that are produced by a great meal or toe-curling sex (which enhance our chances at survival and reproduction, respectively).

Finally, there's a specific quality of bipedal locomotion that appears to be crucial for human development, from infancy on up: something known, again by eggheads, as "contralateral Movement."

Breaking down the Latin into ordinary-speak, we get contra ("opposite") and lateral ("side"). In other words, when we walk or jog or run, we move opposite-side limbs simultaneously.

Right leg and left arm. Left leg and right arm.

Since the two hemispheres of the brain control different sides of the body, the practice of contralateral Movement helps the brain function as a unified whole. This starts long before walking or running: crawling, that first form of human locomotion, is also a contralateral activity. Children who never crawled, or who went through that phase too quickly, often experience difficulties later in life, either related to physical coordination or mental abilities.

Bipedal Locomotion is Not Optional

At the risk of overstating the obvious: walking or running was never a "choice" in our natural, ancestral environment. We didn't wake up and "decide" whether to go to the gym or not. We didn't check our weather apps to see if we wanted to run today.

And we didn't sit on our asses until we found "our thing." You know, like today we try CrossFit, yoga, spin, Pilates, Couch to 5k, and Zumba, lurching from activity to activity until we find that flavor of exercise we instantly enjoy enough to commit to doing regularly.

Your body doesn't care if you "like" running or not, or if running is "your thing" or not. For the vast majority of our time on this planet, life *made* running our thing. As Josh likes to say, you either ran when it was required, or you ended up a lion turd.

And lion turds don't pass on their genes. You are the product of millions of years of evolution of humans who ran when lions were chasing them. Who ran when they saw a yummy antelope. Who walked and jogged while gathering resources for the survival of self, family, clan, and tribe.

So we're not inviting you to "try" bipedal locomotion, to see if it's your thing.

It's definitely your thing. What we're asking is that you decide to DO it.

Just to be really clear, we're not saying that you have to go out and run a marathon this afternoon just because humans are built to run. Or that you have to run at all, now or ever. If you're out of shape, overweight, undertrained, or muscularly compromised, then trying to run would be a crazy thing to do, and would likely result in injury.

But we are saying that you can start where you are, at whatever level of Movement is safe but challenging. Walking, aggressive walking, hiking, jogging, running, sprinting, marathoning, ultra-marathoning — all are valid varieties of this basic human form of locomotion.

Human Movement is Physically Challenging

The second quality of natural human Movement is that it has to be physically challenging. It has to lead to enough stress and system failure within our body that our bodies respond with growth.

There are three physical outcomes that our Movement must create for optimal results: cardiovascular stress, muscular micro-tears, and muscle confusion. Let's look at each one in turn.

Cardiovascular Stress

Basically, cardiovascular stress means our heart rate and the effort and intensity of our breathing rise to a level beyond that of normal life. A stroll around the park or through the mall can be lovely, but if we're not challenging our cardiovascular system, it won't get more efficient, and we miss out on one of Movement's biggest benefits.

Natural human Movement includes daily doses of "hasty." Don't just show up and DO your two miles. Find a baseline for what's sustainable and doable for you today, and move on purpose and with purpose. Spend at least some of those two miles moving at a pace that increases your heart rate and challenges your breathing.

Being out of breath can be unpleasant, especially if you're not used to it. But the wonderful thing about the body is how quickly it adapts to new realities. "Holy cow, that was hard!" our heart and lungs will complain after a vigorous walk or hike. "We'd better get our act together in case that happens again." And that's how we build endurance and capacity.

Cardiovascular disease is the number one killer in the Western world. Challenging your heart can dramatically lower your risk of succumbing to heart disease or stroke.

And we've found that when you build up your physical heart, you also support your metaphorical heart. You feel better, which makes you kinder and more inclined to help others. And your increased capacity for exertion gives you the ability to be more available and powerful when others need your help.

Muscle Micro-tears

Our muscles are pretty remarkable things, when you think about it: the more we stress and challenge them, the stronger they get.

You can't make your house stronger by smashing the walls with sledgehammers. You can't get less breakable dishes by tossing them into the fireplace. You can't improve the performance and longevity of your car engine by racing it twice a week.

But if you tear down your muscles, they just come back stronger and more resilient.

You don't get this benefit by staying in your physical comfort zone. You get it from working your muscles beyond what they're currently capable of. When you do so, you're literally damaging the muscle fibers. Some wisdom in your body then figures out that the muscles need to rebuild stronger.

It's like they reason, "Well, we clearly weren't up to that challenge. And the next challenge might be even worse. Let's grow some strength here."

That's why there's no such thing as "maintaining" our fitness levels. We're either challenging our muscles to grow stronger, or they're moving toward atrophy. We can go forward or backward, but we can't stand still.

The idea of "maintenance" leads to ineffectual plate spinning. We waste time calculating exactly how hard we have to work out to not lose fitness, and in the process accomplish nothing of value.

The understanding that we're either breaking down muscle so it can rebuild stronger and better, or we're not, allows us to focus on progress, which is so much easier to pursue than keeping the status quo.

Muscle Confusion

Along with stressing our muscles, we need to keep them on their toes. The fancy physiological name for this phenomenon is "muscle confusion."

We achieve muscle confusion by varying our workouts. Even if our daily run is cardiovascularly challenging, and tough enough to lead to micro-tears in our running muscles, if it's the same exact workout every day, our body adapts and our run loses some of its value.

That's why you see people who are at the gym all the time but haven't lost an ounce since the first Clinton administration: they've just been doing the same routine for years, mindlessly going through the motions while they focus on TV or music or audiobooks.

Again, let's come back to NAQ. How much of our lives in our natural state would be routine, and how much would be unexpected? A lion wouldn't have said, "OK, I'm about to chase you for 50 yards. Ready, set, go." You would have had no idea how far, how long, or how fast you may have had to run at a moment's notice.

You didn't know when you'd need to climb a tree, swim a river, or fight a wild boar. Life has always been the ultimate in cross-training. Now that we sit for a living, we have to mimic the unpredictable nature of life's physical demands by incorporating muscle confusion into our workouts.

When I (Josh) played football in high school, Coach would have us do these killer workouts. We'd finish up with our wind sprints and then head to the locker room to shower and get our well-deserved rest.

A few times, when we had our pads off and were close to puking, and it was time to go into the field house to get showered up and go home, Coach would give us a speech. "When you're tired like this in the fourth quarter, and you're really beat down, and the offense fumbles the ball right after we got off the field, are you going to quit? Are you going to give up?"

Naturally, we would tell him what he wanted to hear. "Of course we're not going to give up, coach."

"OK, then. Pads back on, and everybody back on the line."

We would have to start a whole other series of sprints—right after Coach had mentally let us off the hook.

That's what muscle confusion is to me. It's what allowed us to beat better, stronger, more talented teams who never practiced digging deeper than they thought they could.

And it's what allows us to rise to life's challenges even when we can't predict when they'll hit us, or how hard.

Here are some simple ways to get muscle confusion into your workouts:

Vary the workouts

Some days are for speed. Some days are for distance. Some days are for terrain (hills, trails, grass, asphalt). Some days are for intervals (hard, easy, hard, easy).

Cross-train

Run. Walk. Do yoga. Perform bodyweight exercises. Swim. Tax all systems.

Try new things

Say yes to novelty and challenges. Try doing a race you've never done before. Sign up for a class that looks weird.

Improvise

Our bodies contain lots of wisdom about how they want and need to move. Feel like doing some dirty dancing? Tai chi? Walking across the living room in Down Dog position? Feel the familiar thoughts of inhibition ("That's silly!"), and then DO it anyway.

Stress/Recovery Cycle

We don't build strength and stamina and capacity while we're training. We build them during recovery from training.

Any Movement is a form of stress on the body. Stress has gotten a bad name, but it turns out that the reality is much more nuanced than the "stress will kill you" message we get from the media and well-meaning but ignorant health professionals.

Stress is a good thing; it forces growth. (Remember micro-tears — they're a form of stress upon the body.) In fact, not enough physical stress makes us weak and sick. Our immune system gets bored and starts attacking our own body through auto-immune diseases, the way a lonely puppy starts chewing on shoes and furniture.

The problem comes when stress is chronic, and never lets up. Mental stress becomes chronic when we're always ruminating on our past failures and future threats, and don't know how to unplug the mind.

And physical stress becomes chronic when we don't allow our bodies the time and nutrients they need to heal and repair following a strenuous workout.

So how do we know how long to recover from a workout? From experience, and from paying attention to our patterns and results.

That's why it's so useful to think of yourself as an athlete in training: if you're consistently improving, that's pretty much proof that you're recovering sufficiently. If you find yourself "working" harder and harder – that is, higher perceived exertion – and yet your performance is getting worse and worse (slower, weaker, etc.), then you have a strong clue that you're overtraining.

Good training builds capacity. Undertraining and overtraining drain capacity. You'll find your sweet spot through trial and error, through action and attention to outcome. And you'll constantly tweak your routine as you grow and change.

Hard is Relative

One of the themes of Big Change is that you have to choose Hard. Uncomfortable. Sometimes Painful (in a good "boy am I sore" way, not in a "I just blew out my knee and can't walk for six months" way).

Just remember that Hard means *hard for you.*

Don't compare your Hard to anyone else's. We're all different. We're all on different journeys. We started at different times and move at different speeds. If you're in third grade, be the best third grader you can be. Don't try to skip ahead to graduate school just because you think it's a better place to be. You won't benefit. You'll likely become bored and unmotivated, you'll probably fail, and won't even have recess. Where's the fun in that?

The only place you can start is Exactly Where You Are.

Don't try to start where you aren't. Don't try to start where you used to be, if you have "glory days" in your past. Don't try to start where you wish you were now.

The only way to achieve Big Change is to become good buddies with Reality. And reality is that you have a threshold of Hard that is unique to you. If it's a 23-minute mile, and you wish you were doing 8-minute miles, then congratulations, you've mapped out the road ahead. Make a plan, work it, and use the Results Dictate Sufficiency engine to determine if you're moving in the right direction.

Human Movement is Wholistic

This might seem obvious, but our ancestors didn't do bicep curls or leg presses or lat pulldowns. They engaged in full-body activities — running, jumping, climbing, pushing, pulling. When they lifted a rock, they used literally every muscle in their body, from the small stabilizing muscles around the feet and ankles to the large muscles of the thighs and mid-back and shoulders to the tiny muscles of the forehead and eyes.

Contrast this with the mechanistic model of most gym weight rooms, where you stabilize the body while working out one specific set of muscles. The problem with this is that you have theoretical strength, but it isn't available to you in the real world. You may be able to curl 190 pounds while your butt is supported on a bench and your upper arm rests on a padded surface, but if you try to lift a 190-pound rock you may pull your back out or strain your neck badly.

Rather than pursuing the unachievable complexity of trying to work all muscles groups equally one at a time, stick to natural, full-body activities as the bulk of your Movement protocol.

Getting Started

OK, so we've gotten the theory and basic principles out of the way. Now it's time to DO something! In this section we'll cover how to get started with Movement in a safe, sustainable, effective, and ultimately rewarding way.

We'll look at the first steps you can take to begin to build a Movement habit, regardless of how "sluggish" you feel right now, and how many New Years' Resolutions to "get in shape" you may have blown off in the past.

We'll look especially at strategies and modifications for folks who are starting with a lot of excess body fat. Josh has been there, and so have many of the folks he's coached in the Missing Chins Run Club (check out their story in *Runner's World* magazine at SicktoFit.com/chins if you could use a shot of inspiration right about now). These tips may save you a whole bunch of blood, blisters, and boob bouncing.

Finally, we'll come full circle and talk about how to balance Movement and Menu, so you don't end up falling for the "Hey, I just burned enough calories to eat a Snickers bar" fallacy.

First Steps

I (Josh) did a whole bunch of things wrong, and a whole other bunch of things right, when I added Movement to my "get in shape" protocol. My biggest mistake was not paying attention to Menu right away (though I got to that eventually, after stalling out following a 100-pound weight loss). And I made others, when it came to Movement. But I want to talk about the Movement stuff I did that worked, so you can model my effective strategies and avoid my idiotic ones.

Aim For a Safe and Gentle Beginning

The biggest thing to remember in getting started on Movement is to start as safely and gently as you can, especially if you are starting cold. Have faith in your (body's) ability to make progress, and know that if you just start DOing the thing, you'll increase your capacity and performance and weight loss and all the other positive outcomes you want over time. It's physics, not faith.

I was a football player in high school and college (until I got hurt and flunked out in the middle of my freshman year—just to keep you from thinking I was some kind of big shot at University of

Arkansas at Monticello), and so my natural domain was the weight room.

I saw myself as a big, strong guy, so I started with what I knew. And it worked, at first. The pounds started melting off, and I was comfortable enough with the scene and knowledgeable enough about the equipment to stay safe and DO the right things.

My point here isn't that you should start pumping iron, but rather that you should start somewhere comfortable. If you used to be a dancer, find some dance classes or dance-inspired fitness classes. If you've always loved the water, then find a pool for some laps or water aerobics. If you feel like the furthest thing from an athlete, then default to our natural human Movement protocol: bipedal locomotion.

Remember, you don't need special gear, or shoes, or clothes, or electronic trackers to go for a walk. You just need to move your body from place to place. If you're in a wheelchair, go for a "roll" instead: use your arms to move yourself around. Just start exerting a little bit more than you're used to, and guess what? You're a human athlete doing what comes naturally.

Once I'd found a good groove, it was much easier to start – slowly – expanding into new types of Movement. After a few months of familiar and comfortable gym training, I realized that my weight loss had stalled and I needed to try something different.

I started sneaking out of the "manly" weight room into the "ladies section" of the gym with all the cardio machines. It took me a while to get familiar with them. I started doing research, beginning with the stacks of *Runner's World* magazines in the gym itself. I slowly worked my way up, starting with running at 3.5 miles per hour for just a few minutes at a time. When I got tired or sore I'd switch to the elliptical machine for a low impact, more intense workout. When I got tired from that, I'd press the Stop button to stay safe. Then, after I'd recovered, I might jump back on the treadmill for another short session.

At 320 pounds, I discovered that five miles an hour would overheat the treadmill motor, which would then shut off until it cooled down. "At your weight," the gym owner helpfully confided in me after the third such stoppage, "the trick is to stay under five miles an hour."

Gee, thanks.

So that's how I ended up walking, jogging, and running outdoors. It wasn't a natural progression so much as a limitation of the damn cheap machines in the gym. No matter — it turned out to be the best thing that could have happened. One mile at a pace of 20 minutes per mile turned into a 15-minute mile, then 13, then 12. Over time, gradually, I got faster and faster, and could sustain it for longer and longer.

True, I pushed myself in just about every workout, well past my comfort zone. But usually I didn't push myself past physical safety. Sometimes I overdid it, but the more experience I had, the smarter I got. I learned how to find that sweet spot between too much and not enough effort, and generally erred on the side of staying safe. The cost of taking it easy one day was minimal compared to the cost of overdoing it and injuring myself.

Start Keeping Records

You'll notice that I was able to speak with some specificity about my progress. That's not because I'm Rain Man. No, I just kept records.

It's not like I became a mad scientist, scribbling furiously in a lab notebook and poring over spreadsheets. I just used my phone to track my workouts.

At first, I tried a bunch of different bicycling and running apps. Eventually I settled on Strava, the social media platform for athletes we mentioned in chapter 2, because of the social aspect. After I got serious, I got a Garmin GPS watch that synced with Strava on my phone.

Even if you don't think you'll need the data when you write your book (and believe me, at 420 pounds I couldn't have imagined anyone ever wanting to know my opinions on fitness), there are several immediate benefits to keeping good records of your training and your results.

Record Keeping as a Training Aid

Having records of my early efforts allowed me to track my progress. When I made progress, I'd gain confidence and my motivation would increase. When I didn't make progress, I would change something and see if that helped. The data was like a GPS keeping me on track, telling me when I was headed in the right direction and when I was off course.

Progress Versus Oscillation

Keeping records and reviewing them on a regular basis trains our brains that the thing we are measuring is important to us. So when you keep records of your progress in Movement, you're telling yourself that getting better is important.

That's especially important if your initial reason for a Big Change is to lose weight, or get off meds, or stop the pain. Those are all "avoid a negative" reasons.

Avoiding a negative can be a very powerful motivator for change; most of us will do just about anything to get out of pain or reduce the risk of something that scares us.

The problem with this kind of motivation is that the further we get from the negative outcome, the less hard we try. Think of it as running away from someone who's chasing us. We run fastest when they're really close, and slow down when we think we've gotten away.

That's why the last 5 pounds can be the hardest to lose. We think, "Well, I've already lost a lot of weight, and that piece of pecan pie looks so delicious."

When we chase a positive outcome, on the other hand, the closer we get, the more motivated we are, and the harder we work. To see this phenomenon in action, go stand at the finish line of a marathon.

You'll see runners who have been limping for the past seven miles suddenly find their stride again when they see the finish line.

Making performance, rather than reduction of suffering, a primary goal means that you achieve progress rather than getting stuck in a yo-yo pattern. Instead of easing off the accelerator as you lose weight or achieve better labs or reduce medications, you keep chasing that goal until you achieve it – at which point you'll be hungry for the next goal, the one that used to seem unattainable.

Personal Pride

I cherish the record of my early runs the same way you might cherish a child's first piece of artwork (especially if that child went on to become an accomplished artist later in life).

Now that my improvements come slowly, in tiny increments, based on lots of hard training, it's nice to be able to look back and see how far I've come. When I'm discouraged at my lack of current progress, I can see those early slow miles and grin at what and who I've become.

So if you're just getting started and you're embarrassed about your current body or capability or situation, start keeping records anyway. Someday you'll look back at the present moment as the low-water mark of your journey. Your future self will thank you, not only for recording this moment, but more significantly for undertaking the journey in the first place when it was uncomfortable and challenging.

Also, don't underestimate those records' ability to fight that persistent Inner Bully that uses any opportunity to make you feel bad in the hope that you'll give up.

Some day in the future, you'll have a lousy workout. You'll feel slow and sluggish. You'll miss your goal. You'll re-pull a muscle that you thought was all healed. And your Inner Bully will have a field day, trying to turn your head into a disco of unworthiness. That's when you can turn to your records and recall, "I've come a long way."

Get lost, Inner Bully. I got facts on my side. You've got nothing.

Your Records Can Inspire Others (and Bust Their Excuses)

Also, as you undergo your Big Change, you will naturally attract the attention of others who desperately want what you have, and at the same time don't think they can get it. They'll look at you as someone "different" and "special" — a defense mechanism so they don't have to face the fact that you DID something to earn that result, and if they want that result, they'll have to DO something too.

Having records of your initial efforts will be inspiring for others. They'll realize that, rather than being a "totally out of their league" athlete, you're just another human being who finally DID the thing and got predictable results—results that they can get as well.

Find Community

One of the biggest things I did early on to support my success was to find and join communities that supported the person I wanted to become.

Community is the single biggest predictor of behavior. Humans are an extremely social species. Our young can't survive on their own, and our adult ancestors needed other tribe members to find food, keep watch, share chores, and coordinate collaborative activities.

And since we're prone to extreme violence as well as deep affection, we've evolved to pay exquisite attention to social cues. Fitting in was important, since ostracism from the tribe meant death.

So we tend to go wherever the herd goes.

When the herd is out running and eating plants and meditating, that's awesome. But when the herd is sitting on the couch and scarfing Big Macs and playing video games during every free minute — it's time to find a new herd.

Community gives us three valuable things: accountability, support, and role models.

Accountability – having to answer for our actions and their consequences – comes from knowing that others are watching us.

And community is great for this, because when we're part of a community, others *are* watching us.

There are lots of cool behavioral science experiments that show we're most honest when we think we're being observed. Dan Ariely at Duke University showed that people in an office respected the break room Honesty Box more when it had eyes painted on it, or when a mirror was placed behind it so they could see themselves.

There are lots of online communities where people support each other's goals: forums, MyFitnessPal, Facebook groups, and so on. They're all valuable, but Strava holds a special place in my heart because of its focus on accountability: Strava differs from the others in that it records your DOings, not your intend-to-dos.

It's easy to tell a group of people that you'll be running three miles tomorrow morning. You'll probably get lots of kudos and thumbs ups. But you can't expect busy people to check in and hold you accountable for your intentions.

On Strava, you get kudos for what you actually DO, not for what you say you're gonna DO.

Support — as in guidance, advice, encouragement, and the occasional kick in the ass—is the second key benefit of community.

I think of posting on Strava as a waggle dance like the one honeybees do when they return to the hive to tell the other worker bees where the good nectar is. You go out and get a hard run in, and then you return to the Strava hive to let everyone know where you found the good stuff in life, so they can go out and get it too.

The Missing Chins Run Club on Facebook is a hotbed of support. We share advice on details like what kind of running gloves are the best, strategy questions related to racing and recovery, and dealing with frustration, pain, self-doubt, and all the other emotions that us ex-fat guys (and all other humans) experience as we strive to improve ourselves.

Big Change isn't easy. At one point or another, we all stumble. We all succumb to doubts. We all get discouraged and wonder if all the effort is worth it. If we're going it alone, we can wallow in those low places for a long time. When we have the support of a community, there's always someone to lift us up and remind us of what's possible, so we can keep going and return the favor some day.

Role models are the third big thing community provides us. The famous 4-minute mile, which had eluded runners for as long as we've kept records, was finally cracked by Roger Bannister on May 6, 1954. Within the next year, dozens of athletes also achieved that result. Once we know a thing can be done, we can let go of doubt and focus our attention and energy on attaining that thing—and that is what role models do for us.

Rich Roll was my most important role model (my Rich Roll model, hah!) because I identified with his story: a former college athlete who got sidetracked by addiction and clawed his way back to health and achievement. I was doubly inspired because Rich decided to turn his life around on his 40th birthday; I was 33 when I began my journey, so I felt I had a 7-year advantage on my idol.

Scott Jurek, whom I read about in *Born to Run*, made me believe that ultra-running was a thing that humans — and therefore I — could DO.

I follow some of my role models on Strava, and get an inside look at their training efforts and races. Seeing what they can DO inspires me to train harder and smarter.

One of the amazing things about community is that once you're part of it, you get to become a role model for others. I would say it's almost an obligation, because role modeling needs to come full circle in order to be a sustainable force for good. With my appearances on the Rich Roll Podcast, in *Runner's World*, and on national TV, I've become a role model for others who now believe that Big Change is possible for them as well. And now, I'm experiencing the unspeakable pleasure of seeing some of my students become role models in their own families, workplaces, and communities. And so it goes.

Starting with Strava

If Strava sounds like your kind of community, you can get started by going to strava.com and signing up. You can use your Facebook or Google account, or just create a standalone Strava account using your email.

The signup wizard is pretty straightforward. The most important thing is to find friends to follow, and people who will follow you. That's how Strava becomes a supportive social network as opposed to simply a place to record your activity. A shortcut is to find a group, like the Sick to Fit Running Club, or another group based on affinity or geography.

We post our walks, runs, swims, spin classes, yoga sessions, and hikes. And we congratulate and push each other, offer advice and guidance, commiserate, and DO all the things that people who care about making each other better DO. Join us!

Tracking with Strava

There are two basic ways to track your efforts on Strava. The first is to download the Strava app to your smartphone. Then just keep your phone on you, and press the Start button when you begin your workout. As long as you're connected to GPS, the phone will keep track of your route, pace, and a bunch of other stats.

If you can't or don't want to carry your phone with you on your workout, you can splurge on a GPS watch. I use Garmin watches. They're a little pricey, but every time a new one comes out, the old ones get cheaper. It's often possible to get nice discounts on older models on eBay, too. You can learn about which one is right for you at your local running store, or by asking around.

Connecting your GPS watch to Strava is pretty straightforward. Once it's done, you can set your watch to upload your data to Strava as soon as you finish a workout.

Strava also connects with Facebook. If you like, you can also program Strava to post all your workouts to Facebook. It just depends how much you want to share, and with whom.

Moving When Heavy

We've covered the basics of getting started, finding a community, and using technology to track your progress and connect with others. Now we've got to talk about the special issues and challenges that come with being overweight. If you've got a lot of excess poundage to lose, you're going to deal with stuff that thinner runners won't have to worry about.

A lot of people feel that they want to lose all their excess fat before they start running. And it's certainly possible to lose a lot of weight without exercising, if you're on point with NAQ in your diet.

But I've found that not only is it possible to start moving while heavy, but there are tremendous advantages to doing so. You just have to take things slow, be smart, and be willing to pay some dues up front.

Let's face it — if running is new and unfamiliar to you, you're going to have to overcome a whole bunch of self-doubting mental chatter, as well as physical discomfort. If you're heavier than your authentic human form, you'll have to modify your Movement to accommodate that bulk. But stick with it, and sooner than you think you'll be moving with less effort and more grace.

Compensating for Excess Body Fat

The first thing I noticed when I started running (actually, the term I used was "jiggle jogging") was how much noise my body was making. It was embarrassing — all the clapping sounds of fat bouncing up and down, and of my man-boobs smacking my ribs and each other.

Turns out that symphony of smacking was a good feedback mechanism for keeping my form safe for my weight. As I naturally tried to jiggle jog more quietly, I stayed slow to reduce the wiggling and jiggling. I found my feet landing as softly as possible beneath my hips, which I achieved by taking short steps instead of long strides.

My brother Dustin, who was even heavier than I was, started jiggle jogging too, and we invented a life-hack version of man-Spanx, wearing a slightly-too-tight undershirt underneath our regular t-shirt to compress the fat and keep it from flopping too much.

But there was only so much we could do to mitigate the early discomfort. You can't help but experience more nagging pulls and tears and inflammation and aches and pains when you're carrying hundreds (or even dozens) of extra pounds.

Hell, it hurts just to live in that size body, let alone exert yourself in it.

But that's why running (and by "running" I mean walking, strolling with purpose, jiggle jogging, and all that) is so important at the beginning. Precisely because it feels sucky, the fact that you're sticking with it teaches your brain that you are serious, and that you are reinventing yourself as an athlete, as an ex-fat person.

The inertia you have to overcome at the beginning of your Sick to Fit Journey is greater than anything you'll encounter later on. When you get over the initial challenge, you've pretty much got it made.

What you don't want is to "waste" that effort by remaining a "big runner" for the rest of your life. I've seen lots of people take up jogging, but never progress to the point where it gets challenging. And so despite spending hundreds of hours on the treadmill or running up and down the street, they never lose weight.

Remember the Results Dictate Sufficiency engine. The result you're going for is reclaiming your authentic human form and using it as nature intended. If your version of running isn't helping you to shed pounds and increase your capability, then you have to be willing to increase the intensity, frequency, or duration of your runs. The pain and discomfort are nothing compared to the joy you'll feel when, in the words of philosopher Brian Massumi, your body assumes "a posture that intensifies its powers of existence."

That may sound vague and weird, but I swear you'll know it when you feel it. It's when you can jog without stopping to rest, when in the past you had to stop and walk some of it. When you can power up a hill and still have energy at the top for a Rocky dance. When you can feel the athlete that's been trapped inside you begin to stir and assert its desire to celebrate the joy of Movement.

Slow is Good

When you're heavy and first getting started, there's absolutely no rush to increase your speed. If you're tracking your progress with a watch or an app, you shouldn't, at first, be pushing yourself to competitive miles or 10Ks. You're just establishing a baseline. And the slower you go in the beginning, the more impressive your later progress will be. So savor the first few weeks and months of walking, jiggle jogging, and easy intervals.

How do you know if you're going fast or hard enough? Your body will tell you.

Are you sweating a bit? Is your heart rate elevated? Is your breathing getting faster or does it feel more labored?

Good! That means you're now using your body the way it was meant to be used, before spreadsheets and meetings and 2-day free shipping.

I originally started speeding up not because I needed to achieve a new personal record or qualify for a race, but because walking started to feel too easy. It was no longer challenging. Instead of plugging in headphones and distracting myself, I started moving faster, to get back to the level of Hard that walking had been when I began.

Chase the right level of Hard, not a particular pace or outcome.

Pain is OK; Damage is Not

When I wrote the first draft of this chapter, I was injured. I hadn't run hard for going on six months - and it was driving me crazy! So I'm writing for myself here as much as for you.

The prime directive on getting started with Movement is this:

DON'T DAMAGE YOURSELF!

If you're injured, you can't train. You can't improve. And you feel like crap. There's the actual pain of the injury, but there's also the insult of suddenly not being able to move, just when you felt like you had something special going. And add on top of all that the shame of having done it to yourself. It sucks.

This prime directive doesn't mean that you should avoid discomfort. You can't make progress without discomfort, and sometimes without a certain type of pain. You'll likely feel both when your Movement protocol pushes you to a new level of accomplishment and fitness.

The key is to get to know your body, and to be brutally honest with yourself.

Dance to the Music Only You Can Hear

I think of the balancing act between not going hard enough and injuring yourself as a dance. The catch is, you're the only one who can hear the music.

What I mean is, nobody else knows whether you actually need to take those couple of weeks off for shin splints, or to avoid reinjuring your ACL (anterior cruciate ligament, a common knee thing), or are nursing a bad back.

Only you can truly know if you're being prudent, or wimping out. Only you can hear the music you're dancing to.

The way you gain discernment on this point is through experience. As someone once said, "You can't know where the line is unless you cross it." So there will be times you will overdo it, and pay with a few days of limited mobility and some pain and discomfort. And there will be other times where you hold your progress back by taking it too easy — by coddling non-existent injuries and playing it far too safe.

What's your default tendency? In the past, have you jumped in all gung-ho, limped home after your first workout, and then spent the next six weeks in traction? Or were you the type who spent 18 months going 1.5 miles per hour on a zero-incline treadmill, making no progress, until you practically fell over from boredom? This is where brutal honesty comes in.

It's a constant set of experiments, this path to knowing your body and its language of GO or PAUSE. And the more you focus on your workout while you're DOing it, the more data you can gather and learn from. I know it's less boring to walk with headphones on or while watching a screen at the gym, but if your head's out of the game, you're ignoring crucial body communications that could guide you to a safe and appropriate level of exertion.

Clues to Damage

There are particular bodily phenomena that indicate the potential for injury; pay attention to these and take them seriously. They include

- swelling (especially swelling of joints that doesn't go down within a couple of hours)
- discoloration (indicating bruising)
- sharp pains that worsen the more you move

If you're experiencing any of these, don't be afraid to find a trainer or a physical therapist who can help you with proper form to help your body heal and prevent future injury.

If you live near a PT who is trained in Total Motion Release (TMR), they can show you some really simple and gentle Movements that can heal and also prevent injury by bringing your body into balance. You can find a comprehensive list of TMR-trained therapists at SicktoFit.com/tmr.

Balancing Movement and Menu

The last thing I want to talk about in the "Getting Started" section is the dangerous and oh-so-common concept that we are exercising *so that* we can continue to indulge with food.

Since the weight loss pabulum of our age is "eat less, exercise more," it's easy to get caught up in the bad idea that we move more SO THAT we can eat more. Lots of runners — even speedy, lean, and apparently healthy ones — express this idea that running "allows" them to eat more, and worse, than if they were sedentary. You see this after races, where finishers drink beer and gobble up pizza that they've "earned" through their efforts.

That's just crazy, to waste all that effort on a momentary dopamine rush that undermines all your hard work. Don't run to eat. Instead, eat to run.

We talked briefly in the previous chapter about the balance between Movement and Menu in terms of NAQ: As a natural consequence of the environment in which the human animal evolved, the more you are able to eat, the more you need to have moved. We needed to walk, run, and expend energy to gather the food we ate, and the more calorically dense that food (for example, meat), the harder we had to exert ourselves to get it.

No other creature thinks about calorie counts, food equivalencies, points, and all that mental nonsense. The squirrel doesn't have to wonder if it's eating too many pecans, because nature has stacked the deck so that the squirrel starves if it doesn't move vigorously enough to gather and store them.

In our natural environment, humans must expend calories to earn calories. And the more calories we want to collect and consume, the more we have to move. This impulse worked perfectly in our ancestral environment, but is a recipe for obesity and disease in a world full of calorically dense, highly processed foods.

I recommend turning the tables on our thinking about the relationship between Movement and Menu. What if, instead of simply thinking about Movement as balancing our Menu, we make

Movement the larger purpose? What if we eat in order to bathe our bodies in nutrients SO THAT we can perform to our greatest potential?

When we avoid hyper-palatable processed foods and limit those from animal sources, we honor our physical journey toward higher and higher levels of performance. If you owned a high-performance sports car, you'd give it the highest grade of fuel possible, right? Your body is infinitely more valuable than any car — so it makes sense to give it the highest quality nutrition.

That's easy to say and put on a t-shirt, but the idea becomes urgent and powerful when we live as aspiring athletes. When we aim not to win races, necessarily, but to constantly make progress. To compete against our past self and consistently strive to surpass what we believed was possible last year, last month, last week.

This relationship to our food is far more empowering than just eating when we're hungry, tired, bored, stressed, or in a social situation that triggers the munchies.

You don't drive your car just so you can fill up with gas three times a day. You fill your car with fuel so that you can get where you need to go. That's the ultimate balance of Movement and Menu. And this is a key attitude to have as you're getting started, to maximize your progress and enjoyment.

Mental Aspects: Staying Committed

Once you've gotten started, the next step is to keep going.

Too often we act like the two Sammies from the old *Saturday Night Live* sketch, who get excited about their new project, but when it comes time to execute, they decide "that's another thing I'm never going to do."

We've all started exercise routines and then watched them sputter and die. We've signed up for a gym membership we didn't use, bought a Nordic Track that ended up a drying rack for laundry, or purchased new running shoes we only wear to the mall. We all know what it's like to start out excited and end up deflated, embarrassed, and ashamed.

Convinced that we're just a lazy screwup who can't commit to anything for the long haul.

The good news is, you aren't a lazy screwup. If you've dropped the ball on Movement in the past, it was likely due to one or more of a small number of avoidable mistakes.

Mental Pitfalls

When you get your mind straight, Movement becomes a lot easier to implement, maintain, and grow. The three most common mental pitfalls that derail a new Movement habit are lack of confidence, discomfort, and stalled progress.

Lack of Confidence

When you think about working out, running, or taking a yoga class, do you ever get the feeling, "There's no way I can DO this"? And that lack of confidence makes you not even want to try?

Both the thought itself and its outcome make perfect sense. According to Albert Bandura, the father of modern social science, the single best predictor of human behavior is self-efficacy: the belief that you *can* DO something.

If you believe you can DO it, you get the opportunity to DO it, and you want to DO it, then you will. But if you don't believe you can, then you can get all the opportunities in the world and you won't take that first step. If you lack confidence in your ability to do something, you can have all the motivation in the world and you will still hold back.

So we've got a bit of a Catch-22 here: you don't act because you lack confidence, and you lack confidence because you haven't acted. What to do?

Simple. You develop confidence in yourself the same way you'd develop confidence in someone else: by giving yourself "tests" to pass.

Think about it — you wouldn't trust every stranger you meet to watch your kids, manage your business, or guard your house. You only trust people who've demonstrated that they're trustworthy through being given, and proving themselves worthy of, greater and greater amounts of trust.

In order to develop trust and confidence in yourself, you have to give yourself a chance to demonstrate what you can accomplish. Start small, but work up to increasingly challenging things. You'll soon see yourself as capable and dependable.

Discomfort

A lot of people start an exercise program and then stop because it sucks. They can't stomach the discomfort, so they fall back into old habits.

Discomfort typically comes in two flavors: physical and emotional.

Physical Discomfort

The physical discomfort we feel when we first start out is all about body aches and pains and other unpleasant sensations such as shortness of breath. It can also include exposure to the elements.

When you start moving vigorously, with purpose, you will definitely experience sensations that you can easily interpret as sucky. Aches and pains, muscle soreness and tightness, gasping for air, sweating like a pig, chafing; these are all common symptoms at the beginning.

A lot of us are also "weather wimps," a condition caused by spending large chunks of time in hyper-comfortable indoor environments at 72 degrees Fahrenheit. So when it starts raining, or the wind is rattling the windows, or the thermometer drops into the 40s or 50s, we find all sorts of excuses to stay indoors and skip that day's workout.

When you add insects, mud, uneven terrain, heat, and humidity to the outdoor exercise experience, you can see why a lot of beginners who try it just give up and go back to their comfortable-in-the-short-term lives.

Realize that we're all different in how heat and cold affect us. You may need to bundle up a lot more than your running buddies. For example, Howard can go shirtless in 20 degrees F, but still has to wear gloves in the low 50s or his fingers stop working.

Emotional Discomfort

Our emotional discomfort at the start of a new routine typically arises from feeling like a clumsy beginner.

When you start something new, you naturally don't know what you're doing, and you can feel foolish. Especially if you're doing that new thing publicly, in a gym or at a running trail in a park, you can feel (or imagine) people watching you, and judging you.

Unless you acknowledge and deal with these thoughts and feelings, they can squash your motivation and send you back to the couch, tail tucked.

One way to overcome this emotional discomfort is through community. When we're part of something bigger than ourselves, we don't feel so alone. Another way is to remind yourself that every expert was once a beginner. And that the You who's starting this journey is braver and more deserving of praise and encouragement than the fit Future You who will reap the benefits.

The next chapter, on Mindset, will give you lots of tools to deal with emotional discomfort without breaking stride.

Overcoming Discomfort and Pushing Through

The reason discomfort stops people is simple: the discomfort is happening in the very real NOW, while the benefits of Movement — of continuing to move despite the discomfort — occur in the theoretical future. Social scientists tell us that we discount the future by 50% or more: we would much rather have $10 now than $20 next Tuesday. And so while we may desperately want to lose weight and reverse disease and feel healthier, those desires compete to outweigh our preference to be comfortable right now.

So what's the secret to overcoming discomfort? It's actually dead simple: enjoy it.

That's right — *start enjoying the discomfort.*

Reframe it in your head. Tell yourself that you're a badass, pushing through this awful feeling to get what you want and deserve.

Embrace the suck. Embrace it big-time.

Tell yourself that everything you've ever wanted, everything that's worth working for, can only be found outside your comfort zone.

Take pride in choosing to feel discomfort. In getting up before sunrise, when the last thing you want to do is leave your warm, comfy bed and go outside in the cold, dark rain.

Take pride in DOing the thing even though you're a beginner — in facing head-on that fear of looking stupid. That fear is just your mind chattering; it means nothing unless you grab hold of it and let it define and defeat you.

Remember that every world-class performer was once a beginner. And that it's the beginner, not the expert, who displays courage and grit as they journey into the unknown. Honor yourself for being vulnerable — for being strong enough to show your weakness to the world, and especially to yourself.

When you embrace the suck and push through your discomfort, you build the most important muscle of all: reality-based self-esteem. You free yourself from relying on other people's opinions of you, and instead build a relationship with yourself.

You start trusting your own word, because you pass harder and harder tests. And even more than that, you start being impressed with yourself. You become your own best friend, your own role model, your own champion.

You start feeling like a team, like a squad, like a gang, all by yourself. It's impossible to describe how good this feels. It's better than any food, better than the warmest, fluffiest bed.

And getting up out of that warm, fluffy bed before sunrise counts as a very powerful fight-thru. Repeat enough times and you build a totally new identity as a person who is true to your word.

A word specifically about nasty weather: it's almost never a good excuse for not going for a walk or a run. Lightning is a good reason to stay indoors. Terrible air quality from smog or a nearby fire is another one. So is air cold enough to freeze your eyeballs, if you don't have extreme gear to protect yourself. Avoid heat stroke and frostbite. Don't damage yourself through foolish and unnecessary exposure to the elements.

But garden-variety cold, wet, windy, snowy, humid, hot, muggy, buggy weather is part of life. Deal with it. And embrace the suck.

Just like the dance between discomfort and damage, navigate the elements with self-awareness and common sense.

In his book *What Doesn't Kill Us*, Scott Carney shares research that NOT exposing ourselves to environmental extremes such as cold and heat actually impairs our immune systems. Without stressors to combat, our immune system can get into all kinds of mischief, which can exacerbate the symptoms of autoimmune diseases.

So don't just tolerate bad weather; celebrate it. It won't kill you, and it will definitely make you stronger.

Stalled Progress

Once we've gained confidence and dealt with discomfort, we may think we're on easy street. When we start moving, it's easy to make amazing progress. Every run or walk is a new milestone: longest, fastest, strongest. The weight flies off, and we feel the difference in our body and our mood.

Then we hit a plateau.

Progress slows or stops. We can't seem to DO our walk or jog any faster. The scale needle feels stuck. We're a third, or a fifth, or a tenth of the way to our goal, and it looks like the end of the road.

So we shake our heads, give up, and go back to our old life and old habits.

We gain all our old weight back, and then some.

Sound familiar?

There are three different flavors of stalled progress. All are natural and normal, and all can be overcome through the right actions and Mindset.

The Natural Plateau

On any health or weight loss journey, there are natural plateaus; times for the body to pause and consolidate.

It's impossible to predict when you'll hit a natural plateau, or how long you'll stay there. But rest assured that you will hit at least one, and possibly several, holding patterns on your way to your ideal weight and fitness level.

The key to navigating a natural plateau is not to worry about it. Your body is much smarter about these things than your conscious mind. The relationship between your day to day actions and weight loss isn't linear. Neither is the relationship between training and improved performance. If you view Movement as a gumball machine that predictably gives you a reward every time you drop a quarter in the slot, you'll soon lose motivation when that formula fails.

Keep DOing. Don't get fooled into giving up, or switching to a ketogenic diet, or any other kind of silliness. Stay the course. The engine of progress will kick on again, and you'll be back on the journey.

The "Where Did Hard Go?" Plateau

The second kind of plateau happens when what used to be Hard becomes easy, and we don't compensate.

Let's say your first effort at a mile took 25 minutes. And you were huffing and puffing and clutching your side for most of the walk, and were sore for the next three days.

After a month, you can easily DO a mile in 18 minutes, feeling fine afterwards. That becomes your new workout. And then you plateau. Weight loss ceases. That 18-minute mile is fine for enjoyment and recovery, but will no longer fuel your progress.

What happened here is that you maintained the superficial details of your workout, but you lost the essence of Hard. You're no longer pushing yourself the way you once did.

If you're maintaining an easy pace, covering the same distance every day, you've adapted. You're now putting in the illusion of effort, rather than truly putting in the effort.

The solution here is to keep chasing Hard. When your existing workout gets easy, ramp it up. Add some short sprints. Increase the incline on your treadmill. Go longer. Add breath holds. Do something — anything — to maintain the level of discomfort you experienced when you were just starting out.

Remember, there's no such thing as maintaining. You're either making forward progress, or slipping back.

Don't ever let it get easier. Just keep getting better.

The "What Got You Here Won't Get You There" Plateau

What Got You Here Won't Get You There is the title of an excellent book on career and personal development by Marshall Goldsmith. As a plateau description, it refers to times when you've made it as far you can on a given protocol. You've adapted, and once the thrill of your current success wears off, you realize that you're stuck. And to get past that plateau, you need to do something different – again.

For example, when you're morbidly obese, those first 100 pounds can fly off from just cutting out sodas, chips, cookies, and donuts, or just walking 20 minutes a day. But once you're down from 420 to 320 pounds, those same strategies will just keep you stuck at your new weight. You've got to clean up your diet even more, or start walk/jogging for 45 minutes a day, to overcome your new equilibrium.

Far from being bad news, this dynamic is one of the most exciting things about the journey. It means that there's always a new level, a new challenge, and an even greater sense of wellness and accomplishment waiting for you. Eventually, you'll look forward to your plateaus. Instead of frustrating you, they'll tempt you with visions of future adventure.

Embracing Your New Identity

The best way to overcome all these mental pitfalls is to embrace a new identity. We know who we are — and by default, what we expect ourselves to DO — based on the stories we tell ourselves about ourselves.

In the old days, psychologists thought that the best way to change our actions was to change our thinking.

Now we know they had it backward: we change our thinking by changing our actions. When we are faced with new evidence, we are forced to reevaluate what we thought we knew about ourselves.

When you go running, it undermines your self-definition as a couch potato. Now embrace that new definition, and cement it in your mind.

Make sure you don't undermine your actions with a bunch of "yeah, buts":

"Yeah, but it was only half a mile."

"Yeah, but I was much faster in high school."

"Yeah, but it was on a treadmill, not the road."

Milk your actions for all they're worth, and actively process them into a new identity.

Actually, your original, genuine identity: Human. Athlete. Runner.

DO. Become. BE.

More Than Calories Burned

In this chapter, we've pushed bipedal locomotion over other forms of exercise. That's on purpose.

To be clear, we've got absolutely nothing against cycling, yoga, Zumba, pickup basketball, or yardwork. We engage in all those activities. (Well, not Zumba. Yet.)

But we're emphasizing the bipedal locomotion because it's the default form of human Movement — it's what humans DO. We walk. We run. We climb up and down. We swim. We lift and carry heavy objects. We cover the ground. We scope out and defend our territory.

Few of us have to DO any of those things in our modern environment. We can get by on swivel chairs, in cubicles, and in the bucket seats of our cars and trucks.

So we have to fit that natural human Movement, natural exertion, and natural exposure to the elements into our lives in an intentional and strategic way.

The goal of Big Change isn't, ultimately, to lose weight, or reverse disease markers. It's to become the best version of yourself. Covering ground vigorously, with purpose, is simultaneously a tool, a metaphor, and a necessary piece of becoming that best self.

Go for it!

Vitamin PD

PD stands for "productive discomfort."

Not the pain of physical or emotional damage, but the discomfort — physical and mental — that comes with embracing a new Movement habit.

We'll be talking a lot more about Vitamin PD in the next chapter, on Mindset. But we just want to add one point here about the benefit of fostering and banking Vitamin PD as part of our Movement protocol: it's highly transferable to other domains of our lives.

Just to give you one example: when you're out with co-workers, it's hard to resist that delicious-smelling slice of pepperoni pizza, and choose a salad instead. Just the idea of it can be daunting.

By contrast, it's much easier to say, "I'm going to keep running for another 20 seconds, even though it sucks."

We can DO pretty much anything for 20 seconds. Or, depending on how awful the thing is, 30 seconds. Or even a couple of minutes.

If you don't believe us, enter a race and see what happens to all your aches and pains when you finally see the finish line.

As long as a commitment is a finite one, we're usually willing to make it. And it's much easier to DO something than to refrain from doing something.

And here's the amazing thing: after we've won a bunch of those fight-thrus around Movement, it starts feeling natural to apply them to Menu — to that slice of pepperoni pizza, or to a Snickers bar.

Once we realize that we're not talking about "for the rest of my life," but only "for now," we can then be present for the food craving in that moment without fear of making a commitment we aren't willing to stand behind. And we quickly realize that our cravings don't last forever, but more like 10-20 minutes at most.

After all, we don't have to resist that slice of pizza forever. Just until we place our order for salad.

We can flex our Vitamin PD muscle, honed during Movement, to help us to ride out the cravings until they subside.

And since it's always "now," we can use this technique to stick to our Menu rules for the rest of our lives.

Get an invitation to join the Sick to Fit Run Club on Strava at SicktoFit.com.

8

MINDSET

The third pillar of Big Change is Mindset. It's less concrete than the other two, but crucial nonetheless. Without the right Mindset, you're not going to maintain the Menu or Movement protocols.

Let's face it: we can give you all the Menu instructions on a Post-It note, and the Movement recommendations on an index card. That stuff is really simple.

But as you know from experience, it's generally not easy.

And because we don't always know how to think about building new habits, we beat ourselves up for making mistakes. We start out all excited, and give up the minute we screw up or our motivation takes a hit. We set vague intentions, and slide away from them without even noticing.

In other words, we don't accept the inevitable, we don't anticipate the probable, and we don't acknowledge the actual.

The Motivation Sustainability Problem

Upgrading our thinking is the ultimate solution to the thorniest problem we face when we try to change our health habits and ultimately, our destiny: that, after a while, our motivation wanes.

One day, we want the Krispy Kreme cruller more than we want a hot body.

One day, we don't feel like getting up early and going for a run.

One day, we're too busy to sit down to meditate.

When we get started, and are totally jazzed, it's practically impossible to imagine that motivation could ever wane. Just like when we're in the midst of a new love affair, it's almost impossible to imagine that someday we'll be annoyed at our beloved for eating all the plums, farting in bed, or using the expensive non-stick skillet as a cutting board.

But trust us: that day will come.

The question is, what will we DO then?

Most people give up on their health and weight goals when they just "don't feel like it" anymore.

When they screw up, they take it as evidence that they're going to fail this time, just like all the previous times—so why keep trying?

They don't think ahead, and so fail to make plans to succeed in difficult circumstances. Then they use the resulting train wreck of a meal or weekend to justify their desire to quit.

Or they decide that the future they dream about is simply not worth the discomfort, inconvenience, and social awkwardness they have to endure in the present.

But you're different.

You understand the whole game here. You're in it to win it. You're no flash in the pan.

Which means that maintaining your new habits is just as important as developing them in the first place.

To make sustainable changes, we have to adopt the right Mindsets. We've already shared a ton of Mindset stuff with you in this book. The FAST Assessment, the pre- and post-mortem, turning a bad day into good data — they have the Mindsets required for success baked into them.

But in this chapter, we'll make those Mindsets explicit. There are three Mindsets that are crucial for long-term, sustainable success: Seek Growth, Embrace Discomfort, and Practice Self-Compassion.

Armed with these Mindsets, you'll be equipped to handle the inevitable bumps, pitfalls, and screw-ups on your Big Change journey and still stumble your way to success.

Success Mindset #1: Seek Growth

If you have a Growth Mindset, you believe that you can change and improve with effort. If you have the opposite, a Fixed Mindset, then you think your abilities can't change, and you're pretty much stuck the way you are.

The distinction was developed by psychologist Carol Dweck, author of the book *Mindset: The New Psychology of Success.*

Dweck argues that a Growth Mindset is the most important predictor of success in school, career, and life in general. While that's debatable, there's no question that people with Fixed Mindsets are way more defensive about themselves, and are more prone to cheating, lying, posturing, and putting others down.

That's because if you can't make yourself better, then you have to resort to making yourself *look* better.

Whereas with a Growth Mindset, you acknowledge up front that you are a work in progress, and you can analyze your mistakes to learn from and hopefully not repeat them.

We operationalize Dweck's Growth Mindset into three parts:

1. You believe you can change.
2. You view screw-ups as learning opportunities.
3. You create fight-thrus as development tools.

Growth Mindset Part 1: You Believe You Can Change

When you have a Fixed Mindset, others' successes just makes you jealous. They don't motivate you to try harder, because what's the point? You aren't going to be able to change.

On the other hand, if you have a Growth Mindset, you'll use the gap between what you can DO now and what you wish you could DO as motivation. You'll seek out true feedback, and use it to improve.

You'll get on the scale and write down your weight, as opposed to hiding the scale under the bed and denying your weight issue. You'll get a physical, so you know your cholesterol, blood pressure, and A1c. And you'll constantly monitor your results and adjust your actions to get you where you want to go.

The best news about Mindset is that we can change our Mindsets. It's very possible to go from a Fixed Mindset to a Growth Mindset — both of us have done it, big time. And it's made all the difference.

You don't have a single Growth or Fixed Mindset – it can vary across different aspects of your life. There are lots of people with Growth Mindsets in the domains of intelligence and skill who still believe that their inability to stop bingeing or to stick to an exercise program are unchangeable character flaws.

Maybe that's you (or WAS you, at this point). You knew that if you studied hard in school, you could improve your grades. You knew that if you practiced guitar, drums, oboe, gymnastics, soccer, or whatever, you could improve your skills. You knew that if you came to work early, stayed late, and requested guidance and support from supervisors and mentors that you could improve in your profession.

But sticking to a diet? "I have no willpower."

Going to the gym five mornings a week? "I'm just lazy."

Meditating instead of mindlessly watching Netflix? "I have no self-discipline."

Can you hear the Fixed Mindset rearing its ugly, disempowering head in those excuses?

So the first Mindset we need to cement to achieve our Big Change is a Growth Mindset around our habits and behaviors. We have to understand that consistently eating right, even in the face of temptation and stress, is a SKILL THAT CAN BE LEARNED AND MUST BE PRACTICED.

We must realize that getting up every day and moving our bodies vigorously when we'd rather sleep in is a SKILL THAT CAN BE LEARNED AND MUST BE PRACTICED.

This is key. Eating right, exercising, meditating, and all that good stuff — they aren't evidence of character. They're skills, just like piano playing or figure skating.

Can you imagine a child taking their first piano lesson and concluding that they sucked and always would, just because they couldn't play Rachmaninoff's Piano Concerto Number 2? Or a beginning figure skater falling down on the ice and giving up because they couldn't nail a Hamill Camel first time out?

Imagine if our schools taught this way. If we thought that first graders should be ashamed of themselves for not already being seventh graders. That high school students should feel inferior for not already knowing what graduate students do. That untenured faculty should regard themselves as forever less capable than full professors.

It's crazy, right?

But it's crazy only because we believe — we know — that each stage is important, valuable, and inevitable. And that by putting in effort, time, focus, and struggle, we can move from one level to the next, and the next, and the next.

That's how it is with health and lifestyle habits too.

We only stall when we stop applying the basic principles of Growth to the task.

Growth Mindset Part 2: You view screw-ups as learning opportunities

The second principle of a Growth Mindset is that mistakes aren't bad. They're our best, most valuable learning opportunities.

In fact, cognitive scientist and learning theorist Roger Schank takes this idea to the extreme: All learning, he explains, is the result of failure.

When we DO something perfectly, we just reinforce our current skill level; we don't get better. It's when we fail and get feedback from that failure that we are able to improve.

When things happen exactly as we expect, we just reinforce our worldview; we don't improve or refine it. When our predictions are wrong, we add new information to our worldview and thus improve it.

FAILURE + FEEDBACK + FOLLOWTHROUGH = GROWTH

So while we don't *try* to fail in adopting new Menu and Movement habits, we nevertheless welcome failure as a natural and necessary step on the path of our Big Change.

Humans screw up.

We are human. Therefore, we shall screw up.

It's not a matter of *if*, but of *when, where, and how.*

Then the question is, "What can I learn from this screw-up that will make it less likely to happen in the future?"

Can you see how different this Mindset is from the one that fears screwing up, because even one single slip-up proves that we're fatally flawed and destined to be fat and sick forever? A Fixed Mindset makes us so fragile that we can't recover from the slightest deviation from plan — even after days, weeks, or months of being totally on point with our diet and exercise.

When we embrace the Growth Mindset, we set our intention to be perfect but realize that we won't be. And that every screw-up holds within it clues to improvement.

Think of shooting a free throw in basketball. When you step up to the foul line, your intention is to swish the ball through the hoop. If you miss, you're not thrilled about it.

You can respond to a miss by beating yourself up for being a screwup, or for choking under pressure.

You can respond by quitting basketball because you'll never be any good.

Or you can respond by noting if the ball went left or right, high or low, then using that information to adjust your next shot accordingly.

And the more you DO that, consistently, persistently, attentively, curiously, over time — the better you'll become at shooting free throws.

Knowing this, you can build your skill by increasing the difficulty and challenge of the shot as you gain competence at each level — from practicing by yourself, to shooting free throws in a game, to being on the line with the score tied and 20 seconds left, to being in the championship game, and so on.

Each new rung on the ladder of difficulty and challenge requires you to learn new skills, new ways of focusing and calming yourself, and new rituals to achieve confidence. But you'll be able to trust that your practice has prepared you to keep climbing.

Once you embrace a Growth Mindset (aka common sense, when you think about it), you can use all the tools we shared in Chapter 3 to get better from these mistakes:

- Post-mortem
- FAST Assessment
- Turning a Bad Day into Good Data

These tools are what to DO, and how to DO it. But the key to actually DOing them is arguing with the voice of the Fixed Mindset that just wants you to quit in despair, and replacing it with the voice of the Growth Mindset that wants you to succeed.

Growth Mindset Part 3: You seek fight-thrus as development tools

The third principle of Growth is to stop fearing challenging situations.

People are scared of — and so avoid — situations where they might screw up. We hear it all the time.

I have to avoid the break room at work because there's always some donuts or cookies in there.

I'm not going to go on that cruise because I'll just stuff myself with crap.

I don't want to have Thanksgiving with my family because I won't be able to resist the turkey and pie.

I'll watch the game by myself so I don't indulge in the buffalo wings and the cold cut platter.

You don't want to put yourself in a situation where you'll fail miserably - that makes perfect sense.

But you also don't want to be OK only in situations that pose no challenge at all, like at home in your room, with only a glass of water and a year's supply of brown rice and frozen kale.

When we rely on our environment to define and dictate our actions, we become extremely fragile. Because we can't control our environment — not completely, anyway, and definitely not all the time.

But we *can* control our own actions. So if want to be in control of our health destiny, we have to put our attention on these areas where we have control, not where we don't.

The more we spend time in increasingly challenging environments and situations, and the more we practice DOing the Menu and Movement and Mindset things, the more "antifragile" we become when faced with the unexpected. With social pressure. With old situational triggers to binge. And so on.

We can make ourselves far more immune to external factors by seeking out opportunities to fail — and succeeding anyway.

That's the whole premise of fight-thrus, which we covered in Chapter 3. Make sure you read that part again, now that you can view it through the lens of embracing growth.

Adopt a Growth Mindset — and practice it, through fight-thrus, again and again and again — and that mental engine will power you inevitably to success. Every single failure will be another stepping stone toward your desired Big Change.

Success Mindset #2: Embrace Discomfort

We've talked about the willingness to endure and embrace discomfort for the sake of our future selves — what we call Vitamin PD — explicitly in Chapter 5, on NAQ, and in chapter 7, on Movement. And we've been alluding to this Mindset throughout the book, on every page, if you know what to look for.

We require Vitamin PD to grow.

In a famous series of experiments, psychologist Walter Mischel gave a bunch of preschoolers a marshmallow, and informed them that if they could wait 10 minutes before eating it, they would be rewarded with an additional marshmallow.

In other words, if they could delay immediate gratification, they'd earn a larger future reward.

What Mischel discovered as he followed those preschoolers over the next few decades was remarkable. The children who were able to delay gratification were far more successful in all aspects of life: career, financial, psychological, relationships, etc.

If we want something in any domain of life, we have to be willing to work for it. To choose an activity that is less pleasurable than some other activity, because the overall payoff is better.

Research Geek Note: Recently some of Mischel's conclusions have been questioned, as other researchers attempt to replicate and refine his work. We don't think the criticisms undermine the importance of our willingness to endure struggle for our long-term success.

Few of us love repetitive practice, or homework, or rewriting, or struggling with something we currently suck at. But those are the keys to getting better at anything. Those are the keys to Growth.

And without cultivating an appreciation of Vitamin PD, we will never reach our potential.

Here are the three things we must do in order to harness Vitamin PD for the sake of our Growth:

1. Accept that discomfort is a natural part of life.
2. Remind ourselves that discomfort is necessary for growth.
3. Choose to practice discomfort consistently.

Accept that discomfort is a natural part of life

In Chapter 5, we saw that physical discomfort is a natural part of life. Humans without access to central heating, air conditioning, and window screens would have had to endure a fair amount of cold, wet, wind, and itching as part of life. Without motor vehicles, power tools, and division of labor, we would be experiencing a lot more fatigue, soreness, and aching as we go about surviving and making a living.

All those sensations are optional in our modern world. But we've made them so at a huge cost.

Here's the thing: pain will find us. Just look at the statistics: people are suffering far too often and dying far too young of heart disease, stroke, cancer, diabetes, and more. These are largely preventable diseases, in most people, most of the time.

Pain isn't optional. It's just a matter of whether we seek it out on our own terms, and turn it into Growth, or whether we wallow in comfort and let pain ambush us through the diseases of its choosing.

We can use pain to become better humans, better spouses, better parents, and better members of our communities. Or we can get used by pain and end up unable to fulfill our responsibilities, and force others to take care of us instead.

We can prevent future pain by choosing some discomfort now.

By eliminating from our diets the hyper-palatable junk that's killing our friends and families.

By choosing to move vigorously, even to the point of discomfort and shortness of breath and muscle soreness.

By withstanding social pressure, and getting made fun of for our dietary choices, and having to deal with people constantly asking where we get our protein, or wondering aloud if we've forgotten how to have fun.

It's not about punishing or denying ourselves the good things in life. Rather, it's about optimizing the whole of our lives, rather than just this fleeting moment.

Remind ourselves that discomfort is necessary for Growth

Let's take cravings as an example.

In the past, you probably gave in to your cravings a lot. Here's the thing: a lot of cravings are triggered by unpleasant feelings that we just want to go away.

Boredom. Loneliness. Fear. Unworthiness. Guilt. Shame. You name it, we try to eat, drink, screw, gamble, work, or Instagram our way out of feeling it.

You now have strategies for dealing with cravings without giving in to them. But we've got news for you: the cravings ain't going anywhere.

You're still going to experience cravings. They might even get more intense, especially when you stop giving in to them. "Hey, if you're not listening, we'll have to shout even louder!"

And you're going to use every tool in your Big Change toolkit to surf that craving until it passes.

When you don't give in to those cravings, you're finally going to FEEL the feelings underneath them. The guilt and shame and frustration and unworthiness and worry and fear and the whole Pandora's Box of ugly emotions.

Guess what? Those feelings suck. They're uncomfortable. They probably feel dangerous, or even lethal. But they're just trying to communicate something important that you're currently ignoring. So rather than resent those yucky feelings and sensations, embrace them as the means to turn you into the sort of person who can tolerate them without needing to numb or distract yourself.

Because, to paraphrase our friend Peter Bregman, if you are willing to feel everything, you can attempt anything. You can grow.

So stay with the feelings. Don't push them away. Practice tolerating them. Listen for what they've been trying to say to you all these years.

All these years that you turned up the volume on sugar, salt, and fat in unnaturally attainable quantities, stuffing your face as a distraction, you weren't allowing yourself to hear and be present for the feelings that needed healing.

Now that you don't use food or other addictions to mask those feelings, you are finally free to experience them fully.

You may need professional help to navigate this part of the journey. If you find that those feelings are more than you can safely handle yourself, then definitely find a smart, committed, qualified therapist to help you get through them safely and productively.

Because here's the true magic of the NAQ diet: not only is it the optimal human diet for health, longevity, energy, and positivity, but by forcing us to face and heal our emotional disquiet, it's also a Yellow Brick Road to Growth.

How cool is that?

Choose to embrace discomfort consistently

Remember, this positive orientation toward discomfort isn't an article of faith, or a statement of character. It's a practice. And like any other discipline in which you choose to excel, you must practice consistently embracing discomfort.

The good news is, you've got opportunities every day in the realms of Menu and Movement.

We're not saying that you can never again eat just for pleasure, or engage in a leisurely stroll rather than a challenging workout. Life shouldn't become a 24/7 boot camp. But pursuing comfort, ease, and never-ending fun in the short term actually diminishes our joy in the long term.

There's a book on parenting with the provocative title *All Joy and No Fun*, by Jennifer Senior. The idea is, parenting can be one of the most joyful human activities. But it's often zero fun. As in miserable.

As in sleep-deprived. As in "I stepped on another frickin' Lego piece in bare feet at 3am on my way to the bathroom."

And yet most parents look back on childrearing as one of the most meaningful and joyful periods of their lives.

Here's the thing: the low-grade misery contributes to the joy. Parenting wouldn't be *more* joyful if our kids obeyed our rules, never acted selfishly or immaturely, and begged for broccoli instead of Lucky Charms. It's the challenge, the effort, the skin in the game that signals to our brains: "This is important to me."

In the same way, we experience joy when we stretch, grow, change, and struggle toward something better, not when we coast in the "good enough" lane.

Joy, as philosopher Brian Massumi writes, isn't the opposite of unhappiness. The two are not even on the same line. Joy can be painful and frightening. Because, at its core, joy is what you feel when you are growing. When you are starting to move toward embodying your true potential, your authentic self.

Joy can hurt. Joy can sting. Joy can cause you to weep uncontrollably.

But ultimately, joy is the emotion of liberation. So commit to practicing discomfort again and again, and free your joy!

Success Mindset #3: Practice Self-Compassion

It's time for an automotive metaphor.

We've committed to growth, to forward progress. We've discovered that discomfort is the primary fuel for achieving that growth. Now we need to mix that fuel with the oxygen of self-compassion to achieve a clean-burning and efficient mixture that keeps our motor in good shape.

Discomfort can easily flip into self-punishment, if we're not careful.

Ever get disgusted at yourself for bingeing, and then go on a fast fueled by self-hatred? Or lift weights heavier and for longer than is good for you? When our minds get hijacked by negativity and self-loathing, we can easily turn the concept of discomfort into a weapon that undermines our growth, joy, and the sustainability of our change efforts.

Enter self-compassion.

Self-compassion is a complex emotion. It's not exactly the same as self-love, although it's close. It's similar to self-forgiveness, but not identical. Educational psychologist Kristin Neff defines self-compassion as being kind and understanding when confronted with personal failures. She has identified three core elements of this Mindset. They are:

1. Self-kindness (instead of self-judgment)
2. Awareness of our common humanity (instead of isolation)
3. Mindfulness (instead of over-identification)

Self-kindness

Say you have a giant screw-up. You eat the world's fattiest hamburger, wash it down with a 64-ounce soda, and finish up with an ice cream sundae.

Once you realize what you've done, you probably gravitate to one of two options. You either mentally berate yourself, or you totally let yourself off the hook.

The first choice, self-judgment, clearly isn't self-kindness. You're just making yourself feel worse, which increases your desire to escape from those feelings with more unhealthy distractions.

But instant amnesty isn't self-kindness either. Most people think that forgiving themselves instantly and moving on is the same as being kind to themselves. But it isn't. You learn nothing from the experience, and so set yourself up to make the same mistake again and again. How is that being kind to your future self, to continue down the path toward weight gain and disability and disease?

But now you know there's a third choice: you can examine your behavior and choices with curiosity and make a plan to do better next time.

True self-kindness is taking responsibility for the future through understanding the past. Instead of shaming yourself for eating ice cream and pie, get curious. Do a FAST Assessment. Collect data. By so doing, you're removing the guilt and shame, and instead focusing on facts.

Armed with that information, you can prepare for the next tempting situation. You can dispute disempowering thoughts. You can create When/Then plans. You can build your capability to resist urges through practice.

Treating yourself like someone who can grow and improve is the ultimate kindness.

Awareness of our common humanity

When you fail, you feel alone. Different from other people, who all seem to have their lives together.

That assessment can lead to a habit of separating yourself from others — from the very people who could otherwise serve as your supportive community. You might think that you don't want to burden them with your problems. Or that you don't want to bring them down with your negativity. Or that they'll judge you and shame you.

Those thoughts are what we call "projections." As in, things your own mind is creating and projecting onto others. Not things that are actually true.

Guess what? We all screw up. We all fall short. We all experience feelings of shame and guilt. Don't believe me? Confide in someone you think is "perfect." Get vulnerable, and share some of your struggles.

I'll bet that they won't respond with, "Wow, you're a terrible person. Get away from me."

Instead, they'll open up about their own problems, shortcomings, and inner turmoil. They'll probably be relieved and grateful that you took the first step in speaking up. And the two of you will get closer.

And as we've seen, being part of a supportive community is one of the best predictors of healthy growth.

Being aware of the fact that our flaws make us more like others, rather than different and separate from them, allows us to see our failings as normal, natural, and inevitable. It takes the pressure off of having to be perfect. It allows us to recover more quickly and gracefully from slip-ups, and increases our ability to connect with others who might support us on our Big Change journeys.

Mindfulness

You can't change what you can't feel.

But if you think you *are* the feeling, you can't change it either.

So there's a middle path here between suppressing or ignoring the bad feelings that come with failure, and totally identifying with those feelings.

That's where mindfulness comes in.

Mindfulness is the ability to be with your thoughts, feelings, and physical sensations without doing anything about them. When you aren't focused on making them go away, you can be present with and curious about them.

And in order to be compassionate with yourself, you must be able to hold that middle ground of neither running away from your inner experience nor wallowing in it. It's not kind to live in a world of make-believe, insisting that nothing's wrong when things are wrong, because you render yourself powerless to change things. And it's not kind to identify so strongly with those feeling that you think you *are* them.

Being mindful about your inner experience does two very important things. First, as you cultivate the ability to stay with unpleasant experiences, you no longer feel as strong an urge to resort to self-destructive behaviors like bingeing to make them go away *right now*.

Second, you're able to learn from those unpleasant thoughts, feelings, and sensations. Have you ever noticed that when you get stressed or feel miserable or depressed, your reactions are way over the top in relation to what's actually going on in the moment? That's because your body is not responding to that moment, but to some past perceived threat to your safety.

When your nervous system gets overwhelmed by an experience, it can get stuck in its response, seeing danger and threat even when none exists. It's like a smoke detector that goes off every time you make toast.

Smoke detectors can't become self-aware and develop a more appropriate response, but you can. Through mindful tolerance and acceptance of negative feelings and sensations, you can actually recalibrate your nervous system and restore it to balance. Then it can evaluate the present accurately, without superimposing the past on it.

It's easier to feel compassion for ourselves when our perceptions and emotions fit life's situations, and make sense on their own terms. We can drop the corrosive rhetorical question, "What the hell is wrong with me?" And through learning about how our nervous system works, we discover that we aren't abnormal or irredeemable, but simply human.

This chapter is all about sustaining your Big Change. Without the right Mindset, all your Menu and Movement efforts will fizzle. When you jettison those old beliefs and adopt empowering ones, you will sustain and build on successes, getting better and better over time.

When you seek growth, you recover from slip-ups and use the data to improve.

When you embrace discomfort, you gain power and agency over your behaviors regardless of the situation you find yourself in.

And when you practice self-compassion, you cut off the fuel for self-loathing that leads to self-harm and giving up.

And you can use the challenges of both Menu and Movement to build that 3-part Mindset of sustainable success.

Bonus Mindset Tactic: Celebrate Non-Motivation

There will be times when your Mindset efforts fizzle as well. When you wake up and feel absolutely no connection to the idea of growth. When you have zero desire to experience any kind of discomfort. When you feel nothing but self-loathing, and self-compassion is the furthest thing from your mind.

There will be days when it feels like the Big Change journey you've been on is over. You gave it your best effort, but you fell short again. Just like all the other times you went on diets or starting exercising, but gave up.

Be brutally honest: you've been fearing that day since you starting reading this book, haven't you? And now it's here. Your motivation has run out, and you don't feel like doing squat.

Now what?

Now you perform a Jedi mind trick on yourself, and celebrate your non-motivation. Or more precisely, celebrate what not being motivated gives you the chance to do.

When that happens — when all you want to do is throw away your food rules, give up on your Movement routine, and stay up all night eating Doritos and watching *The Walking Dead* — that's when you have the most wonderful opportunity to grow and execute the Mother of all Fight-Thrus.

When you DO, not because you feel like it, but because you've decided DOing is who you are and what you DO — your old self will do anything to get you back to that place of easy comfort. It will scream at you to relax, chill out, and give yourself what you "deserve."

You'll be able to hear these voices loud and clear, and you can follow them straight down. Pay attention to what you're thinking and feeling at a time like this. As you begin your workout in spite of totally not wanting to, you build capacity and character and literally change your identity and your destiny.

It doesn't happen every time, of course. You're not demanding that anything happen on schedule; instead, you're continually setting the table and inviting your authentic self to dinner, so that you're ready when it shows up. Then, together, you experience those old patterns and emotions, and can liberate yourself from their influence.

Be Patient

If you've never experienced anything like we're describing here, you may have no idea what we're talking about. If this is totally theoretical to you, and sounds freaking weird, that's OK.

Without a frame of reference, what we're saying is just words. Like if you were trying to explain the taste of a peach to someone who'd never eaten fruit.

The point is, be patient, DO the things, and you'll experience it for yourself.

Be Curious

Also, approach those moments of non-motivation with curiosity rather than anxiety.

Stay light, stay interested, and don't force or resist anything. Just go with the flow, and you'll be rewarded with new experiences, outlooks, and outcomes.

Be Fierce

Finally, realize that in some ways this is a fight for your life. Be a warrior. Brace yourself for battle, and DO your best.

You will actually find a deeper motivation in the center of non-motivation when you remind yourself of the stakes of slipping back into old patterns, vs leaning forward into progress.

9

IT'S YOUR PROGRAM, NOT OURS

T his is the last chapter. You've read it all. We've done our job. Now it's on you.

What are you going to DO?

Despite what the length of this book might suggest, you only have to DO two things:

1. Get started.
2. Keep going.

Use the Menu and Movement protocols to build your own emotional courage and resilience, as we talked about in the last chapter.

A Kaleidoscope, Not a Program

You may have noticed that we didn't include recipes, meal plans, workouts, or guided meditations in this book. We don't believe in giving you "a program." Instead, we believe in you creating your own program, your own protocol, using what we've shared and from everything else that's good and true in your life.

You're going to put it all together like a kaleidoscope. The pieces aren't going to fit together perfectly and they will constantly change. And the result will be messy, and confusing, and non-linear. Some days you'll feel on top of the world, and other days you'll want to quit.

But it will be YOUR program. No one else's rules to follow. No one else to blame if you get off track, and nobody but yourself to get yourself back on track.

We can't chew your food for you. We can't run your miles for you.

All we can do is share our own journeys: that waggle dance bees do to tell their hive mates where the best nectar is.

And be part of your community of supporters, cheerleaders, ass-kickers and guides, if you'll let us.

Limitless: What Else Do I Believe That Isn't True?

Here's what happens when people embark on their Big Change journey: they start out by learning things.

New facts about what foods are healthy and unhealthy.

New facts about why humans get fat, and how we can get unfat.

New facts about how our minds really work, and how we can use them to make ourselves happy instead of miserable.

And once they experience the disorientation that comes from a totally altered worldview, they ask themselves a new question: "What else do I believe that isn't true?"

Then they spend a ton of time UNLEARNING things.

Dropping their limiting assumptions and beliefs about themselves, about the world, about everything.

It's scary on this side of the process, but totally liberating on the other side.

Imagine letting go of all the stereotypes you believe about yourself. All the statements that go, "I'm the _____ one."

The lazy one. The irresponsible one. The happy-go-lucky one. The fat one. The incompetent one. Whatever.

Imagine dropping all those masks and discovering that you've had inside you, all along, a cheerleader, friend, and teammate.

A voice delivering your head and heart a hearty dose of HELL YEAH!

Of quiet confidence. Of self-love. Of deep respect for self and others. Of deep gratitude for all the gifts of this world.

When you let go of how you think things are, then you can observe objectively how they REALLY are.

Welcome to reality. The water's fine. Come on in!

ACKNOWLEDGMENTS

A standing ovation for Leah Wilson, the world's best editor, for giving up nights and weekends to turn our word vomit into coherent prose. To give you an idea of how important she is to the finished product, these are the only paragraphs she didn't have a chance to edit. She would never have allowed the phrase "word vomit" to remain!

Tons of gratitude to:

Olivia Kelly, visionary and CEO of WellStart Health, for supporting, encouraging, and harnessing our wild energy in the service of Big Change in the world. WellStartHealth.com is where the magic lives.

Saray Stancic, WellStart Health's former Chief Medical Officer, and brave warrior on behalf of human wellbeing and sanity. Saray has fought back from a diagnosis of crippling multiple sclerosis, and she's now taking on the medical establishment, working to redefine the practice of medicine from sick care to health care. Her practice website is DrStancic.com, and you can check out her new documentary at CodeBlueDoc.com.

Glenn Livingston, for so generously sharing his *Never Binge Again* methodology with us and with our clients, and for always being good for a laugh. Glenn is also our strategy guru when it comes to coaching, marketing, and life in general. Check out his work at NeverBingeAgain.com.

Peter Bregman, for allowing us to use several of his innovative coaching techniques, including the FAST Assessment. Peter runs one of the most innovative leadership development practices around, and has been a huge source of support and inspiration as we flex our own leadership muscles in the Get Healthy space. Follow Peter (and his awesome leadership podcast) at PeterBregman.com.

Glenn Murphy, science-writer without equal, martial arts instructor extraordinaire, and StressProof ninja, for sharing his insights and and StressProofing exercises with us. Check out his work at StressProof.net.

Tom Dalonzo-Baker, originator of Total Motion Release, for making us smarter, faster, and more flexible in our Movements and our minds. TotalMotionRelease.com is where you'll find details and practitioners near you.

Our Big Change clients, who put their trust in us before we had done anything to earn it. Their faith launched our current trajectory, and made this book possible. Our WellStart Health corporate clients, who are showing the business world that a healthy workforce is both worthwhile and achievable.

Julieanna Hever, Chef AJ, and Tara Kemp for allowing us to use their graphics to illustrate the how and why of a NAQ diet. Julieanna can be found at PlantBasedDietitian.com. Chef AJ tells it like it is at ChefAJwebsite.com. And Tara Kemp inspires and educates at TaraFKemp.com.

Michael Greger, MD, for his guidance about vitamin B12. And for making bright green dress shirts fashionable again! His not-for-profit website, NutritionFacts.org, is the one-stop shop for nutritional sanity and impartial and comprehensive reviews of the scientific evidence.

Clay Garrett for his artistic and design contributions.

Kristin Gara for coming up with the striking cover.

Sue Boyles for designing the spine and back cover.

John Salzarulo for creating the WellStart Health platform and translating our vague wishes into actual website and app features.

The brilliant Yoav Ezer, for guiding us to find a title, and for so generously sharing his strategic marketing brain with us whenever we needed help.

Huge thanks to Patty Hansen, Sue Boyles, Tracie Rheel, Steven Holmes, MD, Nancy Geffken, Melanie Cordes, and Justine Divett for their generous and careful editing of drafts of this book. Every typo, misspelling, and confusing phrase that didn't make it to the page is thanks to them. Every mistake that remains is on we.

Our spouses, BJ (Josh) and Mia (Howard), for encouraging us to live up to our ideals, and showing compassion and forgiveness when we fall short.

ABOUT JOSH LAJAUNIE

Josh LaJaunie is co-founder of Sick to Fit, where he coaches, educates, and inspires people to go from, well - sick to fit. He's co-author, with Howard Jacobson, of *Use the Weight to Lose the Weight*. Josh has been featured in *Runner's World* magazine, *People* magazine, *Good Morning America*, *The Today Show*, and his personal favorite, the Rich Roll Podcast.

He lives in Thibodaux, Louisiana, where he runs miles, eats plants, and beats the drum in his community for the power of lifestyle to trounce chronic disease.

He's also a proud and rabid Saints fan. Who Dat, Baby!

ABOUT HOWARD JACOBSON

Howard Jacobson, PhD, is co-founder of Sick to Fit. He's also the host of the wildly popular (in his home) Plant Yourself Podcast.

Howard is contributing author to T. Colin Campbell, PhD's *WHOLE: Rethinking the Science of Nutrition*, and Garth Davis, MD's *Proteinaholic*, as well as co-author, with Josh LaJaunie, of *Use the Weight to Lose the Weight*. His work has also been featured in Fast Company and the Harvard Business Review online.

Howard is lead instructor at the WellStart Health Coaching Academy, and co-author of the Coaching for Performance chapter of the American Management Association's *Book of Knowledge*.

In his free time, Howard runs, practices Russian martial arts, gardens, and plays far-too-competitive Ultimate Frisbee.

Howard earned his BA from Princeton University, and his MPH and PhD from Temple University.

He lives in Pittsboro, North Carolina with his wife, and sometimes with his adult children. (Fly, kids, fly!)

Printed in Great Britain
by Amazon

25706782R00106